THE POWER OF
ILLNESS

TO CHANGE YOUR LIFE

*A personal journey of healing
and how it can be a blessing*

KAVI JEZZIE HOCKADAY

THUNDERBOLT PRESS

Copyright © 2014 by Kavi Jezzie Hockaday
ISBN: 978-0-9933890-0-9
Published by Thunderbolt Press

All rights reserved. No part of this publication may be reproduced, distributed, or transmitted in any form or by any means, including photocopying, recording, or other electronic or mechanical methods, without the prior written permission of the publisher, except in the case of brief quotations embodied in critical reviews and certain other noncommercial uses permitted by copyright law. For permission requests, write to the author.

The author does not dispense medical advice. Neither does he prescribe any medications for any condition. All information in this book is intended for general guidance only. If you are sick it may be wise to consult your doctor.

Personally I would exercise caution in always going to the doctor.

TABLE OF CONTENTS

Dedication 5
About the Author 7
Preface 9
Introduction 17
What Is the Body? 25

PART ONE - My Story **35**

PART TWO - The Power to Change **91**
Introduction 93
Short Essay on Symptoms 99
Illness Is an Opportunity 105
Healing the Emotional Roots of Illness 115
Cellular Intelligence 127
Cellular Rehydration Through Fasting 137
Clean the Temple 145
Some Words About Raw Food 167
Raw Food Advantages 177
The Ever-Evolving Diet 181

The Problem Is Your Mind ... 187
You Gotta Move ... 197
Living a Noble Life ... 207
Negativity ... 215
Arise Wounded Healer! ... 221
Radical Well-Being ... 227
Conclusion ... 233

PART THREE - Useful Resources ... **235**

DEDICATION

This book is dedicated to my Mother, Louisa Griffiths Hockaday. She sadly succumbed to her illness and it swallowed her up. Her gift to me was both the opportunity to heal my wracked and toxic body and a valuable teaching in how toxic emotions left unhealed ravage and eventually kill us.

It is also dedicated to my wife Amoda Maa Jeevan. She has held me, guided me, supported me, and loved me through the whole journey. Her love does not seem to depend on whether I am sick or well. But she prefers me well! We had no idea that I would get so sick during our relationship, and it was something of a challenge. But her love is so very strong and it lifted me up and became a light to navigate by. She is my muse and my teacher.

Love is such a small word for something that is so vast.

And finally I dedicate this to all those who walk the path of illness. It is tough karma and can be an arduous journey.

ABOUT THE AUTHOR

Kavi Jezzie Hockaday is an Author, Transformational Coach and Musician. After a long and profoundly transformative journey healing inflammatory bowel disease totally naturally, he committed to helping others navigate the difficult path of healing.

He gives talks, coaches others and inspires many. He also plays concerts and writes music.

The focus of his coaching work is giving full attention to his client and developing a true holistic understanding of where they are at and what they want to change. This means sometimes working on the cellular level, looking at diet and health protocols, sometimes focusing in on emotional issues, beliefs and conditioned thoughts, but always considering the spiritual wellbeing of the client. Balancing, cleansing and nourishing the root areas of life can bring about great transformation of the whole.

There is always a movement towards wellness of the organism.

The coaching is tailor-made to the individual needs of the client. This is no 'one size fits all' program.

He loves running, high intensity training, and reading.

He travels globally with his wife and spiritual teacher, Amoda Maa Jeevan.

Coaching website:
http://www.thunderboltcoach.com
Music website:
http://www.kavijezziehockaday.com
Facebook page:
http://www.facebook.com/thunderboltcoach
Skype:
kavijezziehockaday
Amoda's website:
http://www.amodamaa.com

PREFACE

In case you thought, for one moment, that I am a doctor or health professional, nutritionist or homeopath, or some other specialist who can give you specific information about exactly how to cure your illness, if you have one, then I'm afraid I have some sad news for you.

I am a coach and a musician.

I have arrived at this position, writing a book about illness and healing, as a somewhat reluctant author. I have tried to sabotage the experience a couple of times and even told myself it's not my path, and deleted my manuscript. But like an irritating thought that won't go away I arrived back once again with the strongest impulse to share my story and what I have learned. So I have decided, once and for all, to honour that impulse. At least then I can say, 'OK, I have followed through.' This role I find myself in chose me, I did not choose it. I have never met anyone who would consciously choose ten years of illness.

Maybe it is my karma, as they say, that has called me to this journey. Possibly, as John Lennon once said, "Life is what happens while you are busy making other plans."

Or, to put it another way, 'Illness is what happens while you are busy making plans to live forever.'

I certainly wasn't expecting to get sick with chronic illness. I was expecting to live in great health forever until I met my maker, even though all those years ago I was feeling pretty lousy. Actually, more true to say is that, until illness arrived, I didn't give it a second thought. I don't think people who are healthy (by healthy I just mean not ill) do. Everyone is busy living life, and as long as you are moving around and able to get on with it, you are probably not going to contemplate being sick. But the other side of the coin is that you may well 'stick your head in the sand' and unconsciously deny that anything inside you is wrong. That's the breeding ground of illness. In retrospect I would say this is what I did.

Writing a book about illness and healing is not easy. It is a subject fraught with pit holes. There are many experts in every area of health and healing. But you know what? There is always room for one more because between us all we are not doing a very good job! Illness is rampant, and from what I see there are millions and millions of people who simply have no idea that their illness has anything to do with them, let alone imagine they could play any part in healing it. We live in a state of blindness and ignorance, and need as many voices as possible to change this tragic state of things.

What are my reasons for writing this book?

Look around, cast your mind to your family and friends, and tell me, how many sick people do you know? How many sick people who are confused about what to do about their health? How many sick people are afraid of their illness, and even their treatment? How many sick people are afraid to take full responsibility for their situation, turn around and meet everything that being sick brings up, all the emotions and regret and pain and anger and fear? And how many of these people, being paralysed by fear, surrender their own inner intelligence, intuition and motivation to make natural choices, to so called professionals and experts? And just how many people are healed by pharmaceutical medicine? And by healed I mean transformed physically, emotionally, mentally and spiritually? How many people are really able to embrace fully the ups and down of illness, the challenges that come from every angle, and still see the gift in the illness? Not many.

Why not?

Its tough, that is why. There is no map. And it is scary.

That is why I have written this book, for those people.

You see, my contention is that illness can be a calling to transform your entire life. It can be your opportunity to make sense of what might appear to be a meaningless experience. Illness can give our life meaning. It can bring hidden gifts that utterly change the way we relate to others, the world, nature, God, our health, everything. So powerful can illness be that it can change the very way we think about everything!

The Power of Illness

Illness has the raw power to turn us from a fearful, lost, confused, self seeking human being, floundering around on the surface of life, to a brave, purposeful, clear seeing, compassionate, spiritual, healthy, vibrant, service orientated being dancing through life with joy.

Ultimately illness has the power to bring enlightenment. It brings us face to face with death. The transcending of the primal fear that accompanies this reality is powerful beyond measure.

"The more ill I become, the more I see the light in everything." (From the film Winter's Tale *- 2014)*

But it is not only the power it has to transform your life that this book is about. It is also that the process of this transformation brings such a release of energy, such an internal power shift and such a wave of positivity, that it has the capacity to impact illness in a positive way.

This is a two way process, an interrelated movement. The more you open to the possibilities that you are being offered by this new experience, the greater upliftment you will feel and the release of new and vibrant energy will then have a healthy impact on your life.

It can only do this when you meet it consciously. It can only open the door for you. It is you who has to consciously walk through the door and choose, actively, to meet everything that arises once you have stepped onto the pathless path. That is the journey, and that is the invitation of this book.

If you are ill, read this book, it will inspire you to look at your illness again, to look deeper, to ask yourself some questions. Illness is a call to enquiry. It's not an answer, it's a question asked of you at a particular moment in time. And it is a question that is asked over and over again from that moment on. Therein lies one of its gifts. The questions it asks of you get more and more profound and exacting. They change you on many levels of being, not only on the habitual daily level, but on fundamental levels. They ask, who are you really below all the stories? They ask, what is the meaning of your life? They ask, where are you going, what is possible, and what do you believe about healing and health? A thousand questions can arise, and the mystery is not only to answer the questions, *but to live them!* The questions challenge you to live the answers as a new reality, a highly awake and empowered one. If it sounds like a tall order and out of reach, then you are ready to grow!

An oak tree doesn't grow without some discomfort. It has to tolerate all sorts of issues, but it just keeps growing to the light, come rain or shine.

What is this book about?

This book is split into two parts. In Part One I tell my story, giving the emotional roots of my illness, a summary of my life in the 'wilderness years,' and the subsequent arrival of symptoms and illness. I tell how I dealt with it physically, emotionally, mentally and spiritually.

In Part Two I offer you insights into the process of transformation as it relates to being ill. I talk about physical detoxification and cellular health, I discuss the emotional connection as it appears in illness, I talk about developing warrior-like qualities, and I try to inspire you to connect with your innate life force and release it to upgrade your healing. I also include bits and pieces along the way that will give you insight and awareness on the journey.

Who is the book for?

Those who will get most from my words may be ill, but not necessarily so. You will probably be forty-five years old or upwards. This is when we enter the 'danger zone of illness.' If you haven't started having some symptoms by this age then you are doing well, but you may well have, and now is the time to take action. The world we live in, our dietary choices and environmental pollutants stress the body so much that we are less able to withstand the load the older we get. As the load gets heavier, the strength to carry it out of the body gets weaker. Eventually, unless we make conscious changes, we may succumb to the pressure. From approximately forty-five years old onwards through the fifties into the sixties the danger increases.

Of course it is not always going to be the case. Some folk stay healthy their whole lives, but generally they are making good lifestyle choices. The statistics show clearly that heart disease, stroke, diabetes, cancer, arthritis and inflammatory bowel disease all become increasingly likely as we get into our late forties and early fifties. I have recently lost two friends, both in their fifties.

And if you are young and reading this book, congratulations, you have jumped onto the healing path early.

This book is for you if you are on the healing journey and need support and inspiration. And it is for you if you need gentle challenging to take a step further 'out of the box' and make decisions based on what you feel and believe, on your gut instinct, not what others tell you is good for you.

The book has some practical and some inspirational ideas. It is a meeting place of the physical, emotional, mental and spiritual. My hope is that it can support you and inspire you as you dive further into the mystery of transforming illness.

INTRODUCTION

Blowing my Trumpet

I beg your indulgence for a few minutes. I don't often do this but for once I am going to blow my own trumpet, in print, for the world to see.

I have worked very hard to become who I am. When I look back at who I was in 1995 and compare that person to who I am now I can't believe the difference. It's not that I've just matured. Many folks mature but don't get wiser. I seem to have grown in every direction, and the old me seems like a boy, small, unaware, innocent and sick. And I'm not judging myself harshly, that's just what I see, because you must understand I have changed so very much.

I was a tiny seed then. It took major illness to draw the best out of me.

I actually feel like Neo when he was unplugged from the Matrix in the seminal film. The comparison between the man that lived inside the Matrix and Neo that was free and unplugged was indescribable. Chalk and cheese, utterly and totally different, different beliefs, different power, different awareness. I thought I was living life. I believed my thoughts. I had opinions and they ruled my life. I carried a big bag of troubles, some angry, some anxious and many fearful. I was disconnected from my spiritual self and the cosmic universe. I didn't actually have a clue who I was or what I was doing. I was a nice guy, most of the time, but I was messed up emotionally, physically, mentally and spiritually.

And then life kicked my butt hard. And I took notice and jumped at the opportunity. I leaped out of the box that trapped me, went way beyond my comfort zone and burned in deeply challenging fires of transformation. I have worked bloody hard, wept oceans of tears, screamed in frustration and nearly given up many times. *But I've never actually given up.* I lay down once and surrendered my whole life to God. That is different from giving up. Many people know me as a persistent and relentless guy. The memory of being lost in the wilderness for 20 years, and the pain of being housebound for 2 years cuts deep. And so now I can look at everything that has happened and say I have done my time, and 'earned my spurs.' I turned the whole thing around.

I am now here to testify. I'm here to bear witness to the power of the desire for transformation. That desire needs to be overwhelming if it is to carry us through the pain of growth.

> *"Nothing happens until the pain of staying the same outweighs the pain of change"* – **Arthur Burt**

I am here to testify that transformation, although painful and challenging, is worth every tear you cry. Life is not about being comfortable and safe, trying to keep danger and fear out of our experience as long as possible. It is about growth and understanding, wisdom and depth. It's about love and gratitude and compassion. These qualities come from stepping out of our conditioned comfort zone.

I can now see from a 360-degree perspective. The blinkers are off. The anger has gone, replaced with joy. The ignorance replaced with awareness. The fear dissolved and replaced with love. Yes, I am an advocate for transformation, and if illness is what you are being met with, then that *is* your door to transformation. Don't turn away, instead put your hand firmly on the handle and step through. And once you step through, as spiritual teacher **Chogyam Trumpa** said, *keep going.*

The kind of change I am pointing to is vast. It is the end of judgment, the end of identification with illness or pain, the end of identification with the thoughts the ego throws around, the end of anxiety and fear of life or death. It is the beginning of a great peace and joy. It is the beginning of a great compassion and understanding, a vital new view into the heart of being, and an overwhelming gratitude for life as it is. It is the beginning of wisdom and spiritual maturity.

That is my trumpet blown. Thank you for my five minutes of indulgence!

There are some things you need to understand to grasp the depth of what I'm talking about in this book. So let me provide a bit of context. But please remember, I'm not giving you answers, I'm asking you questions. I'm asking you the same questions that were asked of me when I was diagnosed with major disease, and the same questions I have asked myself a thousand times since. That enquiry has led me here writing this for you. I am not an expert in anything other than myself. You are the expert in yourself, but it is up to you to unleash your expertise, your inner knowing. You need to become like the Greek wisdom teachers who said, 'Heal Thyself, Know Thyself.' Right now that expertise may be locked up inside a toxic body, a conditioned mind, addicted emotions keeping you trapped in the past, a long list of medications, or a complete acquiescence to the pervading beliefs of our time.

I really want to help ignite your health and wisdom genius, because by releasing these two incredible qualities you become a powerful force for change in this world. Change begins with you, and your change begins with two areas of your life: your mind and your cells. Get those two things functioning properly and something profound happens.

Toxins in, toxins out? I don't think so

If you imagine for one minute that you are not toxic I invite you to think again. There are people who still think that we can process the crazy amount of toxins entering our bodies easily and naturally. I am not one of them. Toxic load is a big problem for us all, and one that cannot be ignored or swept under the carpet.

Not only are we bombarded from every angle by toxins, chemicals and heavy metals in our food, air, water, household and everyday life products, but our bodies are simply unable to process and eliminate them efficiently unless we actively help them. Some of these toxins our bodies just do not recognise. They completely confuse the immune system, and when the immune system is in doubt, it either attacks or isolates, which means some of these toxins are held in the fat cells until such time as the body works out what they are.

Look at this brief list ...

Chemical toxins: Prescription and non prescription drugs, antibiotics, exhaust fumes, mercury amalgams, pesticides, detergents, household chemicals, bleach, fire retardants, paints, radiation, plastic bottles and products, hair dye, food packaging, airborne chemicals. The list goes on and on.

Electro-magnetic fields: microwave, mobile phones and masts, high voltage cables, viruses, bacteria, fungus and parasites.

Food toxins: Even some organic food is known to contain toxins, and recent tests of some super food and health products has revealed alarming levels of heavy metals and radiation. Non-organic foods are a high risk, not only because of soil degradation but because of the toxins, pesticides and chemicals used to assist their growth. Any processed food at all contains toxins and compounds that insult your liver and threaten your health. But here is the thing about your liver: it is a powerhouse that keeps going no matter what. It will not give you much warning that it is struggling. Alcoholics can keep going for years and years before they collapse. Your liver needs your help as much as you need your liver's help. It's a two-way relationship.

Emotional toxins: Carrying the burden of old, unresolved, emotional toxicity harms the body and compromises the free energy flow, creating weakness and deficiency. Anger, stress, worry, the inability to forgive and let go, holding on to the past and bitterness, are all toxic to the body and need to be released for us to transform our health.

So consider this scenario. You get up after a bad night's sleep with worries about money, angry about feeling powerless, fed up with the past and anxious about the future. You take a shower, wash your hair, put on deodorant, grab cereal and milk, or meat, eggs and bread and jump in the car for work. That sounds pretty normal for some people. But everything you have just done brings toxicity to the body. Toxins in the water you shower in, the shampoo, your deodorant, the bread, the cereal, the meat, and the fumes coming from the air conditioning in your car.

As I have said, some toxins are water soluble and some fat soluble, some the body will release and some it will hold on to. If you are over 45 years old and have never detoxified, you have absorbed a heck of a lot of toxins! And you might not notice the steady accumulation except in very subtle ways. But this is my analogy.

It is like filling a bucket from a dripping tap. One drop is nothing, nor two nor three nor even fifty or a hundred. But eventually after ten thousand drops the bucket starts overflowing. That is called 'chronic toxic load.'

This toxic problem is not recognised and certainly not addressed by modern allopathic medicine, so we are on our own. I'm going to talk about detoxification later in the book.

The modern world will kill us – unless we take action.

For many people these days, illness and disease are inevitable. In many ways it is not so different from 300 years ago, the days of open sewers and poor hygiene, rampant airborne viruses and bacteria. The difference is the cause. But the results are the same. We are in an illness epidemic. Not many people die naturally of old age.

Taking care of yourself physically, emotionally, mentally and spiritually is no longer an optional extra if you want to prevent illness and sustain health. It is an imperative. You will hear me say this over and over again during this book.

My book is about encouraging you, badgering you, persuading you, pleading with you and demanding that you take notice now or very soon, and activate a deeper desire for well being, *whether you are ill or not.*

Motivation

My motivation for health has increased over the years. It began after my IBD (inflammatory bowel disease) burst open and was initially driven by the great desire just to get well and become 'normal' again. After a few years, I realised I would never be 'normal' again and I embraced the journey of well-being and transformation on deeper and deeper levels. Now I am fully committed to constantly upgrading my whole body health and other people's too. I understand so much about the body-mind system that it has made me a servant of wellness for life. It has become a flowing, intelligent, creative, wondrous and mysterious journey into energy. It is so much more than just getting fit or having a healthy diet. Ultimately it is about becoming more and more relaxed and peaceful in my body, and clearer spiritually and mentally. My life is about excellence and radiance in all aspects of being, and embracing all parts of myself, the light and the dark.

So this is my invitation to you. Let us go on this little adventure together. You can have a look into my life and see how much it has changed and what I did to change it. Some of it may resonate, some of it may not. Just enjoy what works and throw out the rest. Remember, all that matters is your journey, and all that really matters is how much you loved yourself and others.

WHAT IS THE BODY?

"The idea that a body can be sick is a central concept in the ego's thought system. This thought gives the body autonomy, separates it from the mind, and keeps the idea of attack inviolate. If the body could be sick Atonement would be impossible. A body that can order a mind to do as it sees fit could merely take the place of God and prove salvation is impossible. What, then, is left to heal? The body has become lord of the mind." - Course in Miracles

"Renew yourselves and fast. For I tell you truly that Satan and his plagues may only be cast out by fasting and prayer." - Gospel of Peace of Jesus Christ

If we could only get this simple question answered all our problems would be solved! But this apparently simple question unravels as soon as it is explored in any depth. I have asked this question over and over again during my long years of healing, I have explored it with my wife who I consider an expert on this subject and even includes a chapter in her book - *Radical Awakening: discovering the radiance of being in the midst of everyday life* - dedicated to the body. And my conclusion is that, if ever there was a rabbit hole, this is it.

First, I would like to tell you a story.

The Land of Forgetting

Imagine ... You are pure consciousness, perfect and formless, surrounded by love and light. Everything is oneness and staggeringly beautiful beyond words. You are united with the most glorious, vibrant soul family. There are no words, no time, no shapes, no form, just utter blissful perfection.

One day you are told that you need to go to a strange land for a while to 'learn and experience.' You are told that you may well forget where you came from and all the love you were surrounded by. You may well forget who you are.

You think that is ridiculous, you could never forget your own true nature, never forget all the love, and never forget the truth of all this perfection.

And then off you go to this strange new land and you arrive excited and wide eyed at the newness of it all. Pretty soon things start happening that create new sensations in you. You have a new experience of yourself and it takes some getting used to. You begin to understand that you are in something called a 'body.' It is difficult squeezing all this consciousness into a small body, but you see others doing it and slowly you get used to it.

You have been assigned a new and very small family and they start to tell you things and treat you a certain way. They give you a new name and start feeding you strange new foods, but mostly they begin to fill you up with all sorts of ideas about who you are and what you are doing there. At first it doesn't make any sense, but you quickly grasp the idea and go along with it. It is easier to copy what you are told than to question things too much.

And as time - a concept you have learned since you arrived - passes, things really change.

You become so attached to the body you have been lent, you actually begin to think it is you. You think you are the thoughts you think, the emotions you feel, and everything you believe. And you totally forget where you came from.

You forget the bliss, the love, the vibration of joy. And you wander around this new place wondering what is missing but unable to remember. You take it all so seriously, as does everyone else.

Your original family know this will happen to you, it happens to everyone who goes to the strange land, and so they send messengers to remind you. But you ignore the messengers and the message. You have totally forgotten where you came from and after years and years of this you are lost. You imagine this strange living is all there is.

Maybe you are sick in this body you have been given? It may seem to be a burden. Maybe you are wounded in the heart and cannot love anyone or anything? Maybe you feel there is no divine presence?

And you are scared and afraid. You don't want to leave. Everyone is frightened of this thing called 'the end,' and do everything possible to prevent it. Life itself seems like a trap. But death is terrifying.

And then one day it is all over. Your journey to the strange land finishes. And leaving becomes very difficult, you have become so attached to it, to the things you have, to the people you know, to the body you live in.

As you leave the strange land something begins to happen. Something inside you starts to remember, and after what seems like no time at all you arrive back to your original home and the waiting and open arms of your ecstatic family. It is wondrous to be back in this bliss!

They say to you, "We sent messengers to remind you, we sent you opportunities to remember. That body you wore on the strange land, you thought that was you. We shook your relationship with your body in the hope that you would seize the opportunity to remember that it wasn't yours! But you just held on tighter and tighter."

And you understood, and liked the game and said, "Can I go back and try again?"

My own understanding of this question has changed many times over the years. I believe it is worthy of exploration before we embark on the journey.

I am indebted to three sources of wisdom: *The Gospel of Peace of Jesus Christ*, *The Course in Miracles*, and *The Transformational Power of Fasting* for my most recent epiphanic understanding. These three monuments of clarity and insight into the nature of the body, sickness, the ego, God and nature, have helped restore faith and calm to a confused mind. I absolutely recommend you read them.

The body temple you have been loaned during your stay on earth has been given by the earthly mother. It is made of the earth, and to the earth it shall return. It is temporary, and subject to natural laws.

Your consciousness is pure spirit. It is perfection, unconditional love, formless and senseless. It is what you truly are, and it is of the heavenly father.

Ultimately all form melts back into consciousness, the formless, which means that form cannot be the master of spirit or the mind. It also means that consciousness and the mind can heal all things, including sickness. This is why miracles can happen.

You are the result of a holy relationship. Your body is of the Earth and your consciousness is of the Heavens. Earth is Mother and Consciousness is Father. Together they create you, and you are the holy child. Your body is the temple you pray in.

> *"God and his laws are not in gluttony and winebibbing, neither in riotous living, nor in lustfulness, nor in seeking after riches, nor yet in hatred of your enemies."* - Gospel of Peace

Like all temples and holy structures, we need to treat our bodies with respect and love according to natural law. Falling out of natural law (natural law meaning a healthy and harmonious, peaceful life) leaves us vulnerable to greed, sloth and sickness. Sin is nothing more than toxic living and an aberrant ego. Jesus associates the devil with unnatural living. When I finally understood that it is not a moral judgement of what is right and wrong, but a question of living according to nature, things fell into place for me. Please understand I am not religious at all. But my search for truth, wisdom and understanding has led me to this deepest of spiritual places.

Unnatural living, what I would call toxic living, is the path of the ego. It is selfish, addictive and all consuming. It has no place for God, is driven by fear and wants everything for itself. It is also the place of dis-ease and sickness. A sick and toxic body is a calling to return to simple living, love, fasting, and nature.

Dishonouring the body temple leaves us empty and fearful, consumed by sin (toxicity) and at the mercy of the devil (our own demonic ego).

Life as we understand it is a harmonious relationship of consciousness and body. When this relationship is toxic and becomes disharmonious, it is a sign that we need to 'cast out Satan.' Jesus preached that we should fast, eat simply, do enemas, and pray. By doing this we eliminate impurities, parasites, fungus and unwanted guests from our earthly temple and restore integrity to the natural system, which in turn allows us to become holy and peaceful once again.

The point here is that in our modern living we have forgotten that our bodies *are* sacred. They *are* the *holy temple* in which we pray to God. There is no need to go to church, you are the church. It is crazy to imagine how disconnected so many people are that they go to their local church, do a few prayers and sing a few hymns and then go to the steak house, drink some beer, insult some driver on the way to the mall and shop all afternoon. Holiness is not an idea or a scripture, it is how we live, the very thoughts we have, the actions we take, the foods we eat, the company we keep, the way we treat ourselves and others. That is holiness and spirituality.

We live in utterly disconnected times.

"God wrote not the (natural) laws in the pages of books or scriptures, but in your heart and in your spirit. They are in your breath, your blood, your bones; in your flesh, your bowels, your eyes, your ears, and in every little part of your body." - Gospel of Peace

The ego will steal everything and claim it owns it. It has stolen your body and has stolen your heart and now holds these things to ransom through fear. Yet in reality all the ego claims is an illusion, albeit a persistent and powerful one. It has the mass of people convinced and running scared of illness and death.

It is very simple. God is love. The Earthly Mother is love. That means you are love. Living as love means honouring the Earthly Mother and the Heavenly Father, which in turn means living a clean, compassionate, natural, peaceful, non-toxic life.

If we have lived a life that has allowed 'Satan' into our bodies and our hearts, then we need to restore balance and remove this satanic influence, which means fasting, detox, natural simple foods and prayer. It is simply that when we are here on Earth we forget who and what we really are, we forget the sacredness of this body temple, and we forget we are holy children walking on the Earth. We forget ourselves as consciousness and take ourselves for our ego. It is a small but terrifying error of identification.

Miracles and Placebos

Placebo effects and miracle healing are proof that anything is possible. They are verifiable proof that matter, in this case our bodies, can be changed by beliefs. Although it defies rational thinking and no scientist or doctor ever wants to discuss it, it is a living reality well-documented that the mind has the capability of healing disease. We live in a world where the common understanding, perpetuated by science and biology, is that most things are fixed in place: A causes b as an inevitable consequence, and once the effect has taken place there is no going backwards. Miracle healing and the placebo effect blow an almighty hole in this belief.

There is a glitch in the matrix of certainty and it is called the placebo effect and miracle healing.

Only quantum science and core spirituality get near to explaining these phenomenon, and they both reveal a world that is beyond the scope of this book. My feeling is that within a couple of decades our understanding of the relationship between matter and consciousness will have advanced so much our current level of knowledge will seem childlike. Great new revelations are coming, and they will reveal such profound possibilities of healing we can only imagine.

Conclusion

Your body is a holy temple lent to you by the Earthly Mother (the divine feminine).

Your consciousness is the eternal you, beyond form or matter. It is what you are before you are born and what you return to when your body dies, and what you are while you are here.

You are a holy child of both the Father and the Mother, and your task is to live a holy and natural life, honouring your body temple and praying to the Heavenly Father.

Most people's lives and bodies have been hijacked by their ego.

Sin, or Satan, is simply a description of a life out of balance with nature.

Sickness is a calling to fast, pray, eat natural foods and cleanse the body back to God.

Placebo and miracle healing is a sign that healing can happen even though the current belief system says it can't.

Anything is possible when we truly believe it.

PART ONE
MY STORY

MY STORY

My Toxic Years

The roots of my illness lay deep in my teenage years. I had a very happy and care-free childhood growing up in the green belt area of Buckinghamshire, United Kingdom. It was the 1960s, and I was young, free and innocent. I played outside all the time and ran crazily among the roaming fields with my brother (two years older) and friends. I thought I was in heaven and life was amazing. I'm not saying everything was perfect, but my childhood view of the world was intact and un-traumatic.

But at the age of eleven we relocated to Kings Lynn in Norfolk because of my father's work. Torn away from familiar surroundings and close friends, the beauty of the fields, and school, I still carry the image of my brother and I peering longingly from the rear window of the car as we drove off to our new life. We left everything behind.

Thus began my loss of innocence. It seems that problems began immediately we moved. We (my brother and I) were not happy in this new place, it was stark and the didn't seem as friendly. Suddenly we just didn't fit kids can be adaptable.

My parents, on the other hand, were not so adaptable, and I can see now all how this move brought all their 'stuff' to the surface.

I think the cracks in my parent's marriage had been around for a while, but in our old life they were hidden under the comfortable surroundings. Now this new and challenging environment, and the stresses and strains that came with it, began to bring these cracks to the surface.

It started as a feeling deep inside me. The ground of my being, this innocent trust I naturally had, began slowly to tremble.

In those days, if you weren't a liberated hippy, you lived in a world of great conformity and taboo. Some things were just not talked about, even in the intimacy of marriage. So if there were problems many people simply didn't have the language to discuss them. Divorce was a dirty word, men would never talk about emotions, talking about sex was off limits and money was something that appeared out of thin air.

I feel some sympathy for people who cannot talk about emotions or discuss relationship problems. I have been there also in some relationships. But if you have children I say this: get over yourself and speak up. Say the truth, even if it hurts or causes embarrassment. Share your life with your child, do not keep them in the dark, it is a thousand times worse. Include them.

So when my parent's marriage developed problems they were woefully lacking in any skills to deal with them, let alone discuss them with us. It all took place in the darkness of avoidance and self-denial. They went through a protracted four year disintegration of their marriage and neither of them could address it or explain it maturely with each other, let alone include us in their troubles. We needed reassurance and all we got was an air of looming trouble.

My life was lived, from age eleven to sixteen, under a shroud of strangeness and foreboding. Something was increasingly wrong but I didn't know what. It was as though the air got thicker and thicker until none of us could breathe. Both my parents became increasingly erratic. My father was withdrawn, uptight and absent. My mother was eccentric and unpredictable. They both began to drink, and the drunken Sunday lunchtime episodes were a mixture of overbearing, crazy and scary.

They were falling out of love, or whatever had held them together, but they simply couldn't face it. He was wracked with guilt, and she carried the rage and fear. (These toxic emotions came back to haunt them in later life.)

By the time I was fifteen years old I had been introduced to, and taken a great liking to, drugs and smoking. It was the early 70's and everyone was experimenting. I was a highly sensitive and vulnerable teenage boy in puberty and developing fast. I was taking the fall from grace of my parents badly, I was obviously insecure and scared, but I had absolutely nowhere to take my troubles. So they lived deep inside me. When I discovered music, hashish, amphetamines, LSD and smoking, I changed almost overnight. I could escape to oblivion and travel to the stars, I could deal with anything and, more to the point, when I was high I just didn't care about anything.

And I rebelled against everything, all structures, school and my parents. My school report and attendance dive bombed in my fifteenth year. It charts my decline very accurately. I had been, until this time, attentive and bright, curious and friendly.

I became wild, and there was nothing my parents could do to control me. I was full of fear, but the fear just lived inside like a festering wound.

Breakdown

My brother and I suspected my father was having an affair but my parents were in such denial it was impossible to know anything with any certainty. We had lost our footing and doubted everything.

And then one day, out of the blue, it happened. I was sixteen. My father arrived home and something in him had changed. He was angry and distant. Only my mother and I were in the house.

He confronted her with such an utter lack of love it stills send shivers up my spine. He announced he was leaving her. He told her, brutally, that she had outlived her usefulness as a wife and a mother. He blamed the whole disintegration on her. My mother, by this stage and after five years of trying to avoid the inevitable, was like an emotional pressure cooker. She was a Scottish woman with a fiery temper but was usually as calm as a mill pond.

Upon hearing these words it was as though a switch had been turned on in her. The lid blew off her emotions and all hell broke loose. She totally unravelled and had what I believe would be described as a classic nervous breakdown. In the ensuing hour or so she smashed up the living room and then attacked me. My father had withdrawn in fear by this time so I was the only target. She ripped my shirts and pulled my hair out, lashing out at me like a screaming banshee. It was terrifying.

Eventually she slipped into a mindless trance as though there was 'nobody home.' She had me in a pincer grip on the sofa. I managed to unravel myself, as one would from a wrestler, and called the doctor, who gave her some sleeping pills and opted to return the following morning. The following morning she was a broken person capable of nothing. Something deep inside had come apart and was in tatters. The doctor returned and asked her if she wanted to leave and take a break. She nodded and within the hour a car had arrived and taken her off to a mental hospital for a 'rest.'

About two weeks later, at sixteen years old, I left what remained of my home. My father had already left and my brother was about to move.

This was the end of my family life, and how the next phase began. I moved into a caravan owned by a farmer's wife who was addicted to prescription amphetamine. The caravan had six people in it, all who were ready to party. I was out of the frying pan and into the fire.

The damage that long period of emotional attrition did to me, the pain of seeing and feeling my father's brutal words, the subsequent meltdown of my mother and the complete disintegration of my once so happy family, I buried deep inside me. I was unable to process it so I buried it. That's what children do to survive. It was my coping mechanism, designed to protect me from destruction. These were the roots of my illness, deeply planted in my subconscious.

From here I dived into a world of hedonism, chaos, abandonment and avoidance of pain, that played itself out for twenty-five years.

The Wilderness Years

Looking back at my twenties and thirties, I often describe my body as a taxi that took me from experience a to experience b. It was just a transport vehicle. I had no conscious awareness, and certainly no love for it, at all. I was a walking mind, hell bent on hedonism and escapism. I kept my body alive but I didn't care how. My twenties were the worst. I took so many drugs I am still shocked to this day. I experimented with all the hard drugs, nearly died from overdose a few times, and habitually used all the apparently 'soft' ones. My drug of choice was 'speed' (amphetamine, whose toxic load buries itself deep in the body). I smoked two packs of cigarettes a day. I ate anything, anytime. It went on and on. I found and chose friends who did the same thing, and we partied most of the time. It seemed exciting and wild.

My relationships, and I did fall in love, were deeply dysfunctional and chaotic. They always collapsed. As soon as a woman got too close to me and stirred up something inside me, I would retreat and freak out. I was a nightmare on the emotional level. I was lost. Any experience that hinted at my early family trauma would catapult me into more traumatic feelings, so I avoided them in favour of drugs, alcohol and oblivion.

In many ways I was just like many young people growing up carry wounds. My story is vivid and dramatic in the telling, but it is the story of many, and many suffer more extremely than me. The sharing of this tale is to show how our emotional wounds and traumas play out on the physical level and manifest as illness unless and until we deal with them.

I had no access to wisdom and no healing outlet for the pain I carried. I was just a young guy, and it was the 80s and the 90s. I put on a good show of being ok, but inside there was a Pandora's box of emotional and physical toxicity gathering in the cells, tissues, muscles and organs of my body.

Volcano Rising

I simmered in this way for many years with only occasional breakdowns. I developed a stomach ulcer, treated with medication, my skin erupted all the time, I had night sweats and my kidneys ached all the time. I passed out frequently. But still I kept going. I was addicted to alcohol, but more addicted to avoiding my pain by any means.

But the volcano was rising and was unstoppable.

My emotional and physical life were seriously unravelling by the time I reached my late thirties. I was alcoholic, but had given up the drugs. I had massive eczema all over my face which brought up huge shame. Under threat of separation from my partner I sought counselling for my alcohol problem as my relationship was coming apart (just like my parents did).

Slowly it began to dawn on me that I had some big problems. My alcohol counsellor suggested I was drinking to avoid pain. This came as a great shock to me, but it opened the first door of understanding.

Fortunately I had been introduced to a shamanic transformation camp in the late 90s, and the experiences I had in that environment began to stir up the pot of my fears, anger and pain. My waking up to the full horror of buried pain devastated me, but it was so deep I still had no access to it.

By 2002 my marriage had fallen apart and the pain in my body was screaming at me to do something. It was a time of great change for me on all levels. I met my now wife, Amoda Maa Jeevan, who was teaching transformational workshops and I joined her as a musician.

She was a health-conscious being who ate well and looked after herself. I was struggling within myself, and meeting Amoda brought the entire story of my life to the surface. She has been the catalyst for my change, and I will be forever grateful to her. Transformation had begun.

Moment of Grace

My life has always been graced. Everything has happened at the right time. There has been an almost mythic flow to it and I feel I have been carried on a wave of personal evolution. The more I have opened to this wave the more grace and love I have received, and the more grace and love I have received the more I open to life. The journey from innocence to fall, to the wilderness years and then the long mapless path to wisdom and healing has almost taken its own course. I have been a willing passenger and player, doing what I needed to do and always saying yes to the journey. I have always said yes to life at important moments.

Ayurvedic Pulse Check

Amoda had met a young couple in London who were training to be Ayurvedic practitioners.

Ayurveda – A brief explanation

'Ayurveda is a comprehensive system of health care that originated in India several thousand years ago. Ayurveda, known as the Science of Life, is as much concerned with enhancing the quality of life and the prevention of ill-health as it is with the treatment of disease. Its fundamental therapeutic approach is to address the root cause of any imbalance, so that symptoms are able to subside naturally, healing can occur and genuine strength, health and vitality develop from within.'

'Ayurveda is firmly embedded in Indian philosophy. However, its principles are universal and can therefore be used beneficially by anyone from any culture, country or climate. According to Ayurveda, physical, mental and emotional health occurs when the three subtle energy forces (known as doshas) called vata, pitta & kapha are in a state of equilibrium. To achieve such doshic balance, specific nutrition, lifestyle, herbal remedies, hands-on treatments and detoxification processes are recommended that gently cleanse and rejuvenate the body, enhance mental clarity and promote emotional balance as well as a greater sense of well-being. More enthusiasm, motivation and creative inspiration are the natural outcomes of this approach.' (courtesy www.ayuseva.com)

This young couple were still in training but took on some case studies to gain experience and real life practice. Amoda was one of those cases. Both she and I knew I needed some help by this time as my body was literally 'boiling' and my symptoms were intensifying.

She asked them if they would see me. They agreed.

Ayurvedic pulse checks are not in any way like western medical pulse checks. They are totally different. Western pulse checks can check one thing: heart rate. Ayurvedic pulse checks can check, depending on the sensitivity of the practitioner, physical illness years before it manifests, emotional traumas in the body, spiritual disconnection, mental issues, fibroids, cancers, blood disorders, in fact all disorders many years before they manifest. Ayurvedic experts say that by the time western medicine diagnoses disease it has already assaulted the body to such a degree that it is very hard to repair.

They detected signs of early arthritis, massive acidity in the body that would lead to inflammation, and levels of toxicity that were critical. Long-term herbal treatment would not touch this chronic condition. They were convinced I needed to take drastic and immediate action to remove the embedded toxins from the cells and tissues of my body or the likelihood was severe deterioration of my health.

They suggested Panchakarma treatment at a clinic in Mumbai, India. I had never heard of Panchakarma and never been to India. We said yes almost immediately. Some answers come quicker than others. But we lacked the resources to go.

Then my mother died.

Mother's Gift

After a radical hysterectomy in the 70s (they were very common in those days, paying scant regard for the consequences) that had a dramatic effect on her hormonal health, and the massive emotional trauma she experienced with my father, my mother's health never recovered. She developed early rheumatoid arthritis, followed later in life by osteoarthritis. By the time she reached her middle fifties her body was wracked with inflammation. It slowly twisted her feet, legs and hands into contortions, grinding her bones together and causing extreme pain. She became known as a classic rheumatoid case in Addenbrookes Hospital in Cambridge and she was shown off to trainee doctors.

She carried so much resentment and rage that she was unable to release. She never forgave my father and could never see him. She was so angry she even tried to get a shotgun from a friend with a view to killing him (it never happened). The pain of this anger buried itself in her joints and tissues. In many healing books rheumatoid is all about anger, bitterness and resentment. Her 'blood was boiling' for years, and it destroyed not him, but her. Inevitably she was placed on large amounts of medication, none of which healed her but pushed the symptoms further inside until they finally killed her. I watched her disintegrate. She was unable to change her diet, and found temporary relief in coffee, sugar and processed foods. She was in and out of hospital for operations as her body broke down. *It was a distressing lesson.*

I have to admit that when I received a call from a paramedic who had been alerted by a personal alarm she carried, and told she was dead, I was relieved. Her pain was agony to witness, and with no end in sight was heart-breaking to endure. So for her to be released from this suffering was to me a blessing. And I had told her I loved her.

I still believe, to this day, that on the karmic level she was teaching me something profound in this life. She showed me what not to do. She showed me what happens when you don't release toxic emotions and you don't forgive and let go. She showed me how these emotions can live in and destroy the body. She showed me that medication does not heal. I received her sacrifice as a blessing and a warning.

And then she blessed me with enough funds to go to Mumbai and have the Panchakarma treatment. I am forever grateful to her.

Panchakarma

We went to Mumbai in the winter of 2004, for a six-week full body detoxification. I had no idea what to expect, I had never done any sort of cleanse, enemas, juicing or fasting. I had never been to India before and so the whole experience came as quite a shock. The details are not relevant to this book, maybe in some future publication I will relate them all, but before we proceed to the events, you need to know a little about Panchakarma.

A brief explanation of Panchakarma:

PK (as it is known) is generally a four to six week process designed to remove toxicity deeply buried in the body, through medicated herbs, deep body treatments, purgation, bastis (enemas), control of diet and rejuvenation. It is designed to rebalance the doshas (pitta, vata, kapha) that are the Ayurvedic descriptions of the body/mind/spirit elements.

The process has been likened to surgical treatment without the surgery. The practitioner who first diagnosed me said it was like leaving the walls of the house intact and removing all the furniture and carpets, allowing the body to rebuild health and wellbeing from the very base upwards. It is a 5000 year old treatment based on the deepest spiritual wisdom, created by the Rishis, India's wisdom teachers. It is an extraordinary process when done correctly.

> *A word of warning. Because of its popularity among westerners there are thousands of places in India that offer Panchakarma. Be wary of some of these. At best they do nothing. At worst they could be dangerous to your health. Always go on personal, reliable and reputable recommendations.*

The PK experience (this first one, I had three in total), was hell for me. It brought up so much fear and anger I found the entire six weeks a complete physical and emotional ordeal from start to finish. I was emotionally and mentally triggered by the Indian style of patient care which seemed chaotic, inconsistent and crazy, but mostly I was triggered by what was happening inside me. The toxins in my body had started to stir, releasing such a toxic headache that lasted the whole time. It was so bad I thought I was going to die. It was like all my hangovers had come home to roost. I felt terrible all the time. Amoda, of course, was fine!

But I just kept going through each phase of the treatment. I do not give up, nor do I blame the treatments. When I do something I always commit to it and see it through. This is what happens in PK. Just stay the course, no excuses.

So this is the process:

Phase one – ingesting medicated herbs and ghee (clarified butter), body treatments, massage, oils, saunas. The purpose here is to loosen up the body inside and out, to soften tissues and organs and to encourage the release of toxins.

Phase two – purgation. This is when things really get going! A mixture is taken in the morning and within an hour or so the body begins to release. For some people this is an easy process, for others it is difficult. For me it was the latter.

Phase three – healing and cleansing enemas to remove stirred up toxins. Phase three is somewhat unpredictable as it depends how sick you are and how much toxicity you can let go of. Phase three continues for quite some time.

Phase four – This is the after-care process and is vital. For at least six weeks the patient would follow a healing diet and take herbal medications called 'rasayanas' to nourish the body on the cellular level.

Of course it was all very dramatic for me, and the doctors were quite concerned, particularly during the purgation phase. I just couldn't let go of all this toxicity. The body will only release what it is ready to let go of, no more and no less. It won't let go of all the toxins in the body at once when it has built itself around them for years. It's physically impossible. And the relationship between body and emotions suggests that the body will only release physically what we can let go of emotionally. I wasn't ready to let go of everything.

The Perfect Balance

There was a pivotal moment that happened one day, one of a few epiphanies that have happened to me on my healing journey. These epiphanies have guided me and deepened me and shown me the way when I needed to be shown. They are, to me, grace showing me the way or telling me to keep going. They lift me to a higher level of seeing and shake me to my core. They have been the driving force of my healing. This was my first.

During the entire six weeks of my Panchakarma I was completely distressed and out of balance. Except for one day.

At some point during the roller-coaster ride, and I don't remember where I was in the treatment, I woke up feeling great. I felt grounded, fearless, clear seeing, level headed and emotionally balanced. It was such a relief and such a revelation. I was shocked by the new and unusual relaxedness I felt. But I was so calm even the shock just melted away. Even Amoda noticed (with some relief I can tell you - I was insufferable and complaining most of the six weeks!).

"Why was this?" I asked.

The doctor had the answer: "This is the first time you have been in balance," she told me, "Pitta, vata and kapha are all in balance. This is how you could be and what you should be like all the time. This is your natural state."

Wow! I was shocked to discover that this feeling of being at home in myself had been totally 100% absent since I was a child. It had a profound and instantaneous effect on me, and turned me into a servant for life. It gave me something to navigate towards. To have a visceral, full body, emotional, mental and spiritual experience to guide me was such a great epiphany I felt blessed and I vowed to seek this wholeness as a permanent state.

And then the next day it was gone and I was back to the headaches and fear and distress. The balanced experience was a memory, and it would take many years before I fully realised and inhabited that state again.

The Dam Burst

Returning from India I really believed that I had solved my health problems. I thought I had unravelled and healed twenty-five years of toxic living in one short Panchakarma. How naïve I was!

> *The roller coaster had just started, it was time to hang on while the ride really got going.*

Symptoms Emerge

Two months after we returned I began to notice blood in my stool. First there was just a little, then more, and then lots more. It was accompanied by a kind of sticky mucus

I had never seen before. I started to feel uncomfortable in my intestines, bowel and whole digestive system. I felt sick and anything I ate triggered a bowel movement. The number of bowel movements steadily rose. I tried ignoring the whole thing but it just got worse. I began to feel terrible and I was becoming very scared. It was time to see the doctor.

There are two important points to make here:

1. What had actually started here was that my body, triggered into action by the Panchakarma, had begun releasing toxins and shifted into healing mode. Actually there was nothing wrong at this point but everything was all right and just needed to be supported. Our culture of disease mentality and ignorance of the body's intelligence labels this as disease and tries to control and suppress it at exactly the time it needs supporting.

2. I do believe, in hindsight, that the cleansing action of the Panchakarma and release of toxins was too fast. Sometimes detox can happen too fast and the body cannot handle it. This may have been the case, we will never know.

The doctor immediately referred me for a colonoscopy (camera inserted into the bowel) to look for any signs of problems.

I attended the University College Hospital in London for the examination (which is invasive but not traumatic and quite easy).

And then I had to wait for about four weeks for the results to come through. Those four weeks were a kind of limbo for me. I knew nothing about bowel issues or diseases although I had previously had irritable bowel syndrome (I now feel that was an early warning sign), and I was out of my depth. I was in fear by this time. I had witnessed my mother's downfall and did not want to experience anything remotely like it.

I 'googled' my symptoms and can only advise people against doing the same thing, it just triggers horror stories and the worst case scenario outcome. Don't google your symptoms unless you are prepared to be very scared! It is better to deal with reality than the thoughts of a scared mind.

So I went away, alone, to a friend's house in the country to contemplate my situation and wait for results. The week or so I spent alone really did something to me that prepared me for my meeting with the consultant. I wept for what I had done to my body and my life, and what might happen. I was full of remorse. I broke down and broke open. I allowed myself to feel terrified and alone and to surrender to the possibility that this was very serious and I might die. I didn't deny any of these thoughts and feelings, yet neither did I build a big story of poor me or victimhood about it. It was real, it was happening, I was scared, I might be seriously ill. OK now what?

That stood me in good stead for the results.

The Consultant's Office

I went alone to the hospital for my results. It was something I had to do myself, to face this alone. By this time I was as curious as I was scared. I had experience of Ayurvedic and Chinese medicine and homeopathy, all of which I trusted and I knew western medicine was not particularly trustworthy with chronic conditions, so I was cautious. I didn't realise how powerful this meeting was going to be and I certainly didn't expect it to propel me into a journey that would last ten years and take me to every hidden part of my being. I was not prepared for what I was told or my decision, but it was an extraordinary moment in my life and another truly epiphanic experience. I am still grateful for the unfolding of these perfectly timed events.

The consultant was, as you might imagine, serious, professional, formal and businesslike. He 'cut to the chase' immediately. "Mr Hockaday, you have a particularly serious case of **inflammatory bowel disease**. We are not sure exactly what type but we are pretty sure its **ulcerative colitis** and possibly **Crohn's disease**. It is serious and needs urgent attention. I suggest we put you on anti-inflammatory medication right now and possibly steroids to 'get it under control.' But make no mistake, you will have this now for the rest of your life. If the medication doesn't control it, we may have to perform surgery to remove some or all of your colon and replace it with a colostomy bag. This is common procedure for this type of disease."

I recoiled as though I had been hit three times. I heard 'major disease,' 'have it for life' and 'colostomy bag.' The rest was a blur... bang, bang, knockout.

But I didn't lose my composure or inner strength. In fact his words woke me up. I have many weaknesses, but I am also tenacious and not easily bullied or overpowered. I sensed something was drastically wrong with this picture, I just didn't trust what he was saying, and I certainly wasn't convinced by his authority or his jargon. I opened up a dialogue and tried to have a conversation with him. It didn't get very far. "We don't know what the cause is, it just seems to happen to some people."

"Do you think it's got anything to do with diet?"
"No," came the kurt response.

And that is the moment I became deeply unhappy with what was happening. Even in my naivety I guessed diet would be related to intestinal problems. That is not rocket science.

Here I was at a crossroads of my life, a serious life changing moment, and I felt as though I were, to put it bluntly, a set of symptoms with a personality. He didn't see a living, breathing, human being who was scared and looking for answers. As far as he was concerned he knew the truth and I didn't, and that gave him power. He was the expert and I should do as prescribed. He was right and I should not ask too many questions. But the truth was I was seeking answers on a deeper level than he was able to give me, so our conversation was going nowhere.

My heart goes out to those who are diagnosed with cancer or other extremely serious disease and they are blessed with an unsympathetic consultant. It must be very painful.

I attempted to promote and discuss the benefits of the natural healing methods Ayurveda and Chinese medicine with him but it fell on stony ground. He thought Chinese medicine was dangerous and he warned me strongly against these 'alternative and untested' methods. I sat stunned by his arrogance. It was intense and we were at an impasse.

And then it struck me! I could sign myself out of their care and go it alone. Genius! I became animated and almost happy by this revelation and I announced it to him. He argued against this (what he saw as) stupidity, but reluctantly gave me the forms to sign with the agreement that if I didn't succeed I could return for the treatment. I will never forget his final look at me: 'You will be back' it said.

I have not seen him since.

As I walked through the hospital heading for the exit something inside me had changed. I had experienced some sort of awakening, and even though I had just been given the bad news of a serious diagnosis, I was excited about the utter mystery that was about to unfold.

I looked around me as I fled the hospital. Everyone looked sick, not just the patients, but everyone. There was a vibration of sickness, a resignation to disease. *The sickness seemed to be a sickness of the soul and the mind, a sickness of knowledge and awareness.* Nurses, doctors and patients alike looked resigned to the drama and helplessness of the process of disease. There was no sign of health anywhere. The café was full of sick food, there were many people, staff and patients, smoking, there was just no vibrancy or optimism or love or joy anywhere. It was depressing and I felt ill just being in the place.

I was glad to get out and rushed home to tell Amoda my exciting and scary news.

The Long Road of Healing and the Forest of Shadows

This is where my story really begins. But a word of explanation for those readers expecting a 'how I healed ulcerative colitis' or 'how raw food healed my disease' book. I am sorry to disappoint you but this is not a 'how to' book. I have said this before and I want to repeat it often.

This is a 'why to' book. I have observed many people who have been very sick, both my parents, and many clients and friends. When we are faced with a diagnosis, each of us has a choice. That choice is constantly with us throughout our life. It is the choice of *how we meet our experience*. It may be one of the only real powers we have, and the only one we can hang on to during the journey of our lives. It can be deeply challenged by sickness, by death, by all manner of horrors, yet there it is as a choice we always have. It is the ultimate freedom taught by spiritual teachers.

And yet most people live in such a conditioned state they are hopelessly unaware they even have a choice. They easily become victims of life. They are programmed to respond in a robotic way.

Inevitably some people choose to go down the natural healing path and explore themselves emotionally and spiritually. Some heal their illness, but all of them heal their emotional wounds. They all heal some aspect of themselves because their why was big enough. Others resigned themselves to their fate and lost their power, and their lives. For me, giving up to the system that I didn't trust was not an option. I'm not completely against all medical intervention, in fact at times it is vital and life saving. But this 'one size fits all' approach needs to be tempered with wisdom and awareness, and a holistic understanding of the whole person. I did not get a sense of that depth of understanding, so I rejected it. These were intelligent, well educated people. So why were they so lacking in holistic understanding?

Why weren't they looking for the cause of my illness, and addressing that?

The Long Road of Healing

Even my Ayurvedic doctors were shocked by this explosion of what was being called ulcerative colitis. It came like a flood as the dam crashed open. It was relentless and unstoppable, and during the next few years it opened the door to every fear and every suppressed emotion I held in my body. It became a whole person experience, fear unleashed in the body, emotion and mind. And I was utterly lost with it. Looking from now in 2014, back in 2005 there was precious little information on natural options on the internet. So I felt quite alone and in the dark. But I knew things had to change.

I refer to the next five or so years as the walk through the forest of shadows. This metaphor stuck with me as it describes accurately how frightening, mysterious and lonely it can be. It is dark, and behind every tree is another shadow. The shadows seem real, but in the light of day they all disappear. The dominant emotion is fear. It is hard to see the light but slowly, if you place one foot in front of the other, you see it in the distance. That light is your call to healing. It may be physical healing, or emotional or spiritual, but the light symbolises healing. If there is no light, even the faintest light somewhere far away, then there is no hope, and without hope there is no positive energy, and with no positive energy it is very hard to heal.

Never doubt the power of the mind in activating healing. In fact without activating your mind healing may not be possible.

I was trying to hold on to my life but in truth it was falling apart, and calling me to go in a different direction. My body was demanding more and more of my attention and would settle for nothing less than 100%. I had no idea it was going to dominate my entire life for the next ten years.

Ulcerative Colitis – a brief description:

UC (as it is known) is actually what it says, ulcerating and inflammation of some, or all, of the colon. Any disease that has 'itis' as a description involves inflammation. To be precise, this is just a description of a set of events happening in the body. It is not a disease. There is very little consensus in the medical world as to why it happens and that unfortunately means they cannot treat it at its causal level.

If you can't find the cause you can't heal the illness.

The symptoms of UC are: blood loss; mucus; many uncontrollable bowel movements per day (I reached about 20); severe and debilitating cramps and gut pains; bloating; anaemia; malabsorption and malnourishment; weight loss; anxiety, fear and depression. Some people have such serious 'flare ups' they need to go to hospital. It is a chronic condition with acute episodes and periods of remission. Some experts believe it is an 'auto-immune' disease whereby the immune system begins to attack the body, unable to differentiate between friend and foe. Candida and leaky gut are linked to UC.

Unlike other so called 'diseases,' digestive and bowel inflammation is tricky because of the constant impact of food and fecal matter moving through the system and interrupting healing. The system never gets a rest. If I knew then what I know now I would go straight to a water fast, but I knew very little at the time. And I was very weak.

Let me just repeat this one more time. The medical world cannot heal this condition as I was told. In fact they do not believe it can be cured or healed. They explain having no symptoms as 'a period of remission.'

It is also thought that there can be a continuum process if not addressed that runs:

IBS (Irritable Bowel Syndrome) > IBD (Inflammatory Bowel Disease) > Colon Cancer

I believe I was lucky to have had the dam burst open when it did. This traumatic but necessary experience unblocked the colonic build up of debris and fecal matter that could result in colon cancer. It also began the process of releasing the toxic build up in the tissues and cells of my suffering body.

Between 2005 and 2008 I returned to India twice for two more Panchakarmas. Any more would have been ill advised and even dangerous, but they seemed like my only option to remove the toxicity that was at the root of my problems. These two cleanses left me emaciated, fragile and nutrient deficient. I was delicate, easily stressed and had no core strength.

Dropping Everything

When we returned from the final Panchakarma in August 2008 we left London and our urban life (we had both lived in London most of our lives) and moved to a poorly converted barn in Somerset, deep in the countryside. We had, by this time, collapsed Amoda's teaching and we were both on a voyage into the unknown, me physically and emotionally, and her to allow a new and deeper purpose to develop (she was already writing her book 'How to Find God in Everything' by this time)…The book has now been republished with the title 'Radical Awakening: discovering the radiance of being in the midst of everyday life.'

Moving away from everything familiar and comfortable and into the unknown and challenging environment of the country compounded my already extreme detoxification process. It took it to another level that included bringing up and looking at every unloved and unresolved part of me. All my fears, anger and self doubt began to scream at me. I will be brutally honest. I was triggered, angered and scared by almost everything. The silence, the noise, dogs barking, our neighbour, our landlord, the darkness, towns, even the local shop! And worst of all, it was cold and damp (and in the long run this fact returned to cause me a few more problems).

I can see now from my current perspective how necessary this part of the journey was. I needed to let go of absolutely everything. In fact I didn't have to consciously let go it. It was taken from me. I had no hiding place, nowhere to go. I was exposed in the face of this thing, and so I was forced to embrace it. And by embracing it I mean I didn't push it away. It would have been easy to go and get medication that would have probably pushed my symptoms away, back into my body. It may have brought some quick relief. Most people would do that.

But every fibre, every cell in my being was saying, 'stick with this, no matter where it takes you, just keep on going.' I listened to that voice, not the voice of the rational mind. I'm crazy like that.

Housebound

From about 2008, for a couple of years, or so I was 90% housebound. My symptoms were severe. If I ever left the house I had to guarantee that wherever I went I had immediate access to a toilet, the urgency was so instantaneous. I was going approximately 15 to 20 times a day and still losing blood and mucus. I wouldn't travel, go out, exercise, work or meet friends. I often felt utterly exhausted and at the bottom rung of the ladder. It was the lowest point of the journey and healthy and being well looked a long way off in the distance.

I no longer thought about being well. I had surrendered to the journey and now it was a case of 'one step at a time.' It wasn't a plan as such, it was just unfolding in this way, and the physical and emotional pain was so strong and relentless I was pretty much on survival mode at this time. There are times when pain and suffering is so acute all plans disappear and we are brought squarely into the moment, living life one minute, one hour, one day at a time. I experienced some of this, but am fortunate that it was not extreme. My heart goes out to those who have to deal with acute pain all the time. That is tough, a real test.

It took all my nerve and trust, and all Amoda's love and wisdom, and of course the help of some healers, to stay the course and not freak out and resort to medication during these dark years.

Nutrition

I had no idea at all what to eat. I couldn't tolerate any food, my colon was on fire and very inflamed, so almost every single food irritated it, caused a bowel movement and more blood and mucus. It is a difficult situation with bowel inflammation because you need to eat, but what you eat makes the situation worse, so you are stuck. We just did not know then about raw food, juicing, smoothies, fasting and super foods or medicinal herbs and mushrooms.

It is incredible to take a step back and see the revolution in natural health awareness and resources that has taken place in the last ten years, thanks to two things, the internet, and the desire of so many to heal illness and pursue physical, emotional and mental excellence. We are in the midst of a wellness revolution, it is an unstoppable and organic movement of very different people and communities with many things in common, the primary being the upholding of natural law that says the body is an infinitely intelligent self healing organism, and when provided with the right support, can make miraculous changes.

But in 2008 I was in the dark ages of my life. I was willing to make changes but had no idea what changes to make. The question asked by so many was also my daily mantra; "What shall I eat?"

So for the next couple of years I struggled through on a basic diet of quinoa, over-cooked and mushy white rice, avocado, steamed broccoli, some tinned fish, Ayurvedic meals, and not much else. I had given up meat, wheat, sugar, gluten, tea and coffee. I often liquidised all my food and drank it. I wasn't absorbing nutrients and, after a test by a naturopath, found I was deficient in many essential vitamins and minerals. Life was touch and go, a kind of hanging on while the body adjusted to the three Panchakarmas and the movement of all those toxins. It certainly wasn't instant healing, it really was like climbing a mountain one step at a time. It was an exercise in the deepest trust and persistence. I was like a child taking baby steps with no knowledge of where the steps were taking me.

Looking back on that period now opens my heart and I am shocked I was so far down the rabbit hole of illness. I was very difficult to be with and it did challenge my relationship with Amoda. She did not sign up to live the rest of her life with a sick, moaning and complaining housebound partner, and although she was committed to our love it did put a stress on her. Partners of those who are sick are often overlooked, yet they often make great sacrifices to care for and love others. This is, for me, yet another reason to heal our lives and heal our health and commit to wellness, it's not just an act for ourselves but also for our loved ones.

In 2010 Amoda made a trip to America. I remember that period well as I pushed her into going alone. Although I have always wanted to go the US, I just felt too weak and sick. I would have been a burden and she needed to 'fly free.' It was a good move and she appreciated it. And while she was away I stumbled upon the growing market of superfoods on the internet. And when she returned (she had been in California) she was raving about the 'raw food revolution' taking place there. The raw food diet was almost unknown here in the UK, even in 2010 (incredible isn't it, nearly everyone has at least heard of it now!)

So we jumped, dived and buried ourselves in this new and exciting world of food. It immediately uplifted me and took my cleansing to a different level. When you first meet the raw food diet, it is a very mysterious and confusing experience. You can be very lost, not know what to make, and feel very alone, as though you are the only ones doing this 'weird food thing.' Pretty soon other 'raw foodies' appear, usually online, and you begin to feel part of something, some movement.

The thing is, the plant-based raw food diet is *very cleansing and very cooling*. It is powerful. It is very fibrous. It is also very challenging for people with impaired immune systems, those with compromised digestive fire, and those who, in the Indian tradition, are high vata (notoriously unable to tolerate cold and raw food as it creates gas, bloating and air that disturbs the body and mind). So this all new and incredibly powerful diet felt great, created excitement and a buzz, but also had consequences, not all good, as you will see.

Healing Crisis

When the beautiful lotus flowers, it is always worth remembering it has its roots deep in the mud. And so it is with us. The deeper we can go into ourselves, the higher we may reach into our wisdom and health. And so my current wellbeing, wisdom and maturity has its' roots in this period of darkness. Everything I felt, did, ate and thought challenged me. I was close to breakdown often, but I hung on by my fingernails and gradually developed the inner qualities of a warrior. I had to, it was the only way to survive.

And I had crisis after crisis that challenged my faith and trust over and over again. Let me give you an example.

Take the Pill? Would you?

I thought I was turning the corner of healing. I had been diligently doing yoga, chi kung, breathe work, relaxation, visualisation, affirmations, a soft and easy diet, supplements, Ayurvedic herbs, and keeping stress-free. Inch by inch I seemed to be getting better, but it was excruciatingly slow. When chronic disease is so embedded in the body/mind system, there is no magic bullet to heal it. It takes time, care and a lot of patience.

One day all hell broke loose. I was bleeding from the bowel like an unstoppable torrent and we were both terrified. It looked as bad as it could get, as though something had ruptured. I got to the doctor who booked me an emergency colonoscopy and advised me to take medication immediately to 'control the blood flow.' This time I was so scared I decided I was going to take the medication, my faith was being severely tested and fear had taken over. I accepted his prescription, went to the chemist, got the packet, went home, popped them open and held the little pink pill in my hand, and paused. I didn't just thoughtlessly swallow it down, I waited and I felt the vibration of this pill (it seems now like something out of the Matrix film). I asked life what I should do.

The vibration of the pill felt cold and lifeless.

And I received a very strong intuitive message in that moment to not take the medication but to trust even deeper the process of healing. Sounds crazy? Well, I listened to that inner voice and I threw away the medication. One day later, all the bleeding had stopped and my healing took a quantum leap forward. That sums up how the healing process can work. It moves forward, it goes backwards, and then it shifts forward again to a new place. To intervene at the wrong point can sometimes set us back on the path.

I am still amazed at how close I came to taking that pill.

*Please note. I am not advising anybody not to take medication. I do not say take or do not take medication. Sometimes it is the only option. I do believe, however, that if you take medication that suppresses symptoms, inevitably you have to heal yourself from the medication AND the illness. I am not anti-medication, I am pro awareness and information. I am a person who advocates following natural treatments as much as possible. Ultimately, armed with awareness and knowledge, it is entirely your choice what you do.

Further Down the Rabbit Hole

It was during this time in my journey I was called to dive further down the rabbit hole and consciously address my emotional wounding and the pain I had buried inside. The natural movement of my life had brought me to this point, and I embraced it.

It was all about the past, and it was my relationship to the past that I needed to heal. I needed to let go of my parents, forgive them, forgive myself, understand why they did what they did and finally drop the story.

Life only delivers us the experiences we can handle, and this was my time.

It was time to turn around and face my family, fully and consciously. I knew my healing would not be complete until I released the pain from my body.

I was fortuitously introduced to a process that helped me dig out the original 'poison' from my emotional and physical body. The organisation likes to keep the details secret so I cannot reveal the name.

Over a weekend 'training' with approximately sixty men (it was only for men) we were challenged, encouraged, invited and persuaded to dig into our emotions and find those places within us in which we had been disempowered and emasculated as men. It was a very powerful experience and one I would recommend to any man.

There was a central process to this experience, and in this process we were encouraged to focus on one particularly traumatic event in childhood that had 'hurt' us the most. It was as though I was in the perfect place at the perfect moment. Other men were reluctant to go into this vulnerable area but I was ripe for the warriors challenge.

What happened was this:

An experienced man stepped forward to play my father. Another equally experienced man stepped forward to play my mother. I played myself, aged sixteen. It was their task to replay, as authentically as possible, the moment back in 1976 when my father announced to my mother he was leaving, and she had a breakdown. This was a 33-year circle somehow being completed. The atmosphere was electric, and even those holding the energetic space felt captivated. So we tried the first time, the man playing my father announced 'I am leaving you, you have outlived your usefulness as a wife and a mother,' and the man playing my mother freaked out, but it just didn't work. I didn't feel anything, I knew it was just a game. So I stopped it and asked them to do it again, and this time to give it everything, to take it to the top level and make it 100% real. These two guys were incredible and I love them forever. They did.

As the words left my father's mouth and the reached my mother, she/he exploded. As she/he exploded it was as though I had been shot in the stomach. I was physically catapulted backwards and hit the floor doubled up in the fetal position, totally shocked and bewildered.

And then I understood just how deeply the pain of that moment in 1976 had buried itself in my body. It had closed my heart that day and I had lived a life in a state of shock ever since.

This was my return to love.

Emotional pain had become physical toxicity. There was a direct link between the trauma of a wounded sixteen-year old and the manifestation of major disease 30 years later. I was shocked, but wept tears of gratitude that then set me on the road to forgive my father and truly let go of pain.

A little later I took the decision to travel across the country to meet my father, this time not as an angry child berating his guilty father but as a maturing adult who simply wants to finish all guilt and toxic anger and to look him in the eye and say, 'It is over, I forgive you, I understand you were doing the best you could and it's ok.' I needed to do this for me. He received me as well as he could but it was so difficult for him to break out of the guilt that had held him prisoner all those years.

Emerging from the Darkness

Our four years in Somerset in deep isolation were absolutely necessary for my healing to happen. The time, space and the unknown allowed me to dive fully into my healing. I had been to the bottom of the well, touched my core pain and now there were new shoots of growth emerging. I was, inch by tender inch, getting stronger.

There was a momentum to my healing that was both carrying me and demanding my constant active participation. And I was still committed.

Many things began to change. We both started to embrace the raw food diet. I did a lot of juicing and making smoothies. We grew wheatgrass and drank it all the time. I began an online superfood business that gave us unlimited access to a vast array of healing super foods. Amoda published her book and began to find her true purpose as a spiritual teacher. The sap was rising after our deep three-year winter and it was time to reintegrate with humanity.

But healing is not linear. We expect our healing to be on a continuum from illness to health and when it doesn't conform to this mental model we so easily intervene or give up. I was becoming very wise to this error of judgement and am convinced it has saved me on numerous occasions. Healing has never been, for me, a linear experience. It has taken me everywhere: forwards, backwards, sideways and even turned my world upside down. It confounds our expectations and that is where we need to wise up. The wise one knows not to expect a smooth ride. I was, by this time, getting very used to riding the tiger of healing and dropping all expectations. For me, as for so many, the trick is to drop expectations but not to lose faith. Dropping expectations does not mean giving up or becoming despondent or resigned. It is, more simply, dropping our ego's story that healing should happen by a certain time or look a certain way, and when it doesn't we lose heart.

Two Steps Forward One Step Back

Our house in Somerset had been damp and cold, and mould had grown on the walls (this is common in the UK). My immune system was not strong and had been seriously compromised by my health challenges over the years. The cold and the mould were too much for it to handle, so even though my colitis was slowly (and I mean very slowly) beginning to heal, there were other problems manifesting.

The raw food and juicing, although I absolutely loved it and it was my lifestyle food of choice, was inherently cold and cleansing and ineffective at the time at warming up my core body temperature to keep airborne fungus at bay. I contracted fungus and mould in my system during these years and it slowly started to manifest in 2010, three years after we moved there. It didn't leave my system until 2013.

Mould and fungus is a serious and largely ignored problem that should not be taken lightly. It can wreck health and take years to recover. Many houses suffer from it and I always advise people to get a professional mould-check done. Western medicine doesn't want to talk about this problem and hasn't got a clue what to do about it. Even natural healers can find it difficult to diagnose and deal with. But it is a serious and growing problem. I believe I contracted fungus during my time in Somerset and it bedded in due to my ineffective immune system. It began to creep in through my finger nails, but all the time my overall health levelled out and I just wasn't improving.

My circulation was very weak and in winter months I began to suffer from extreme bony chilling cold, the kind of cold that does not respond to more jumpers. Have no doubt, fungus and mould are living spores that will grow anywhere, including the human body. In our fourth year of living in Somerset I lost one finger nail and another one was badly infected. My immune system was so weak I just couldn't deal with the infection so I was forced on to antibiotics, which impacts colon health, which of course impacts colitis symptoms. It was all pretty serious and I was relieved when spring turned to summer and I could get some warmth into my hands.

Keep on Keeping on

We moved to Hastings in 2011, relieved to be reintegrating with society again. It was still damp and cold by the coast and my circulation reached a very low point in winter that year.

In 2012 I lost **5 finger nails**! They fell out, or disintegrated. I had another bad infection on one of my fingers that turned very nasty. Yet again it was a very bad time for me. I was so cold I was scared. I sought tests from the doctors and they revealed Raynaud's syndrome (circulatory issue), probably Hashimoto's (hypothyroidism) and possible Scleroderma (connective tissue disorder). None of the doctors mentioned fungus or mold. By this time I had absolutely no faith left in conventional medicine to deal with chronic disorders, so I wanted the test results and that was all.

I had been researching health and illness, investigating alternative options for healing, asking questions, listening and learning for the better part of ten years and I had begun to understand some fundamentals and key points. I was beginning to join the dots. And what I saw alarmed me.

I saw that our health and our illness was one of the most misunderstood areas of life.

And within that misunderstanding I saw that conventional medicine was as much about business as it was about health and was actually consumed by its own arrogance, dogma and greed. I saw that we are lost in sickness and health misunderstanding on a fundamental level, personally and collectively. I think it was during this time I became committed to helping others to wake up from the dream of what I call *sickness consciousness* and start taking deeper and deeper levels of responsibility for their well being.

I began giving talks about my own health journey, and was interviewed on the radio about what I had learned. It seemed my story gave some inspiration to others who were lost and confused and lacked the confidence to step out of the matrix and turn towards nature. I was shocked by this, and I am still shocked by this.

In 2012 I found a Chinese doctor who was, in my eyes, a master healer. I arrived at his clinic in Hastings UK with terrible circulation, freezing hands and feet, barely any finger nails, bloating and occasional colitis symptoms, and all the disease labels the doctors had thrown at me. He said I had fungus in my system and in my hands that had been growing for a while and had dug in pretty badly. He was practiced in body intelligence and rather than treating me with herbs he began to work on the energy systems of my body through deep body work and chi activation. He also had me soaking my fingers in vinegar every night! I responded very well. I dropped being a 'raw foodie' and ate warming foods, soups, broths and vegetables, even some tofu. I didn't have any meat.

This confusing journey was about to reach a new level of health that has brought me to this table in this moment typing this for you. We are approaching the zenith of our journey, thanks for sticking with me!

2013 - My Best Year Ever!

My health took a quantum leap at about midpoint of 2013. Everything began to come together, and has been on a constant rise ever since. I joined a gym and started work on my core strength and muscle fitness. That had an almost immediate effect of warming me up. My running improved, I was running 15 kilometres by this time with unlimited energy. I was getting up at 5am each day and doing a regular practice of the Tibetan 5-Rites and the gym or running. We went to bed early and rose early, something we had done for years (which really helped stabilise my energy). I adopted a more flexible approach to my diet, responding to what my body told me it wanted. Not my desires but my body. When it was cold, it wanted more warming and sometimes cooked foods, and when it warmed up it wanted high raw. I still live like this today, I found that imposing a diet, any diet, even raw food, on my body, is counterproductive to my health.

My motto is responsible and intelligent flexibility.

I also did a liver cleanse for the first time in 2013 and I honestly believe that helped the leap of health I have experienced. As I have said before, I sometimes wish I had known these things years ago, because even though it has been a perfect journey in its mythical way, I may have saved some time on the health front.

As the year unfolded I felt more and more energy and power. Physically, emotionally, mentally and spiritually life was coming into harmony. My awareness was clearer and clearer. I felt consistently grounded, not like the fleeting moments I had experienced before. I felt better than ever, I felt younger than I had ever felt, I was becoming fitter, smarter, brighter, more open and more enthusiastic, had more insight, clarity and zest for life. I was absorbing nutrients and minerals, my skin looked clearer and my eyes sparkled. Wow!

I had blood tests toward the end of 2013. My thyroid markers were normal. My ESR levels (markers of inflammation in the body) were normal, all finger nails were growing back, I no longer felt cold (well slightly, it is UK)! I had no symptoms of inflammatory bowel disease, and I had no blood, no mucus, no bloating, and no swelling. My bowel movements became good. There was, and still is, a vulnerability in my colon, particularly in what was the most affected side, the transverse colon, and during times of great stress or very late nights, or eating the wrong thing once too often, it will tell me in no uncertain terms to 'back off' and ease up. My wound has become a kind of navigation system. It tells me when I'm on course and off course. I cannot let my desires run amok for too long before I get a message alerting me to the dangers. I don't think this is a bad thing and I appreciate this early warning system.

I was reminded in late 2013 of the time back in my first Panchakarma when I felt balanced and grounded for one day and was told by the doctor that this was my natural state, how I could feel all the time. Well, here I was almost nine years later in the same state constantly.

My excitement and love of the healing process became my life, and my awakening.

Becoming Whole

In 1997 as part of a year of a Shamanic Contemplation course (a profoundly transcendent and transformational experience with a gifted shaman and mystic) I took part in a powerful ceremony that involved climbing the sacred mountain of pilgrimage called Craugh Patrick in Ireland. The purpose of the ceremony was to symbolically cast away part of ourselves that no longer served us. I held a small mirror in my hand that symbolised a negative view of myself I no longer wanted. I climbed the mountain before daylight with the mirror in my pocket and when I reached the top I pulled the mirror out to find it had cracked on the way up. *I looked into it and saw a fragmented reflection of myself.*

So I prayed to God on top of that holy mountain as the sun came up, and I shouted and screamed to make me whole. I took the mirror and threw it with all my might into the abyss, sat in silence and climbed down the mountain. At a talking circle later that day I announced I would give up drinking, a decision that stuck with me until this day.

Sixteen years later that fragmented view no longer exists. It took many years to reassemble my wholeness, but the joy I now experience of feeling fully here and fully whole gives an extraordinary aliveness and energy to life.

And when I had psychosynthesis therapy in 2009 I discovered there were fragmented and unintegrated parts of me that lived subconsciously in the shadows. At certain moments of life, particularly stressful or challenging moments, one of these fragmented parts would emerge and take over the running of my life, usually from a fearful stance. These parts, in therapy they are called sub-personalities, are the carriers of our wounds. When denied or neglected they carry tremendous power and can seriously damage our lives. They contribute to addiction, depression and violence, and are finally only released through awareness, forgiveness and integration. I discovered a very wounded, hurt, unloved and angry 15-year old living inside me who so badly wanted to be seen and loved it was heartbreaking.

Becoming whole is the journey of reintegrating those parts of ourselves previously neglected and unloved, consciously and lovingly acknowledging them as worthy and valued parts of the whole. When the light of love and conscious awareness is shone on these areas of life they become allies and beautiful children. They no longer have toxic power and no longer contribute to illness or the sabotaging of our lives or relationships.

What is denied in one self causes harm to one self.

This integration is a crucial aspect of healing all illness and creating wholeness. It is the root of holism. To be fully healed means you have to address the whole being. Our societies, steeped in traditional science and religion, address each symptom and each illness within the broader context of fragmentation and never attend to the whole. This is, in my view, an absolutely fundamental error of enormous proportions. Our western culture lost the wisdom of the ancient Greeks whose word 'holos' is the basis of our word holism. 'Holism' is considered an alternative idea among mainstream thought and rationalist science. Orthodox medicine considers things as separate. It separates symptoms and tries to deal with them with pharmaceuticals that are isolates separated from nature. The chances of going in to the doctors and them treating you as a whole person, physically, emotionally, mentally and spiritually, are very slim.

And clearly, to these eyes, we can see the results of this separatism. We are sicker and dumber than ever. And generally speaking, the majority of people who are healing their illness, depression, alcoholism and other addictions, are doing so because they address their issues holistically.

From Cells to Spirit

There is an invisible thread that runs from matter to spirit, some may call it consciousness. Everything hangs on this thread, including emotions and thoughts. Matter and spirit are simply different vibrations of consciousness. Gandhi, a well known faster and advocate of simple eating, once said, *"Spirit is matter rarefied to the utmost limit. Hence, whatever happens to one's body must affect the whole of matter and the whole of spirit."*

Understanding this continuum helped me see that by addressing my own cellular health in the early days of my diagnosis and by cleaning up both the cells and the surrounding interstitial fluid, I set myself up for all the subsequent healing. When the cells are healthy, then we also are healthy. There is a connection between the nourishment of the cells and the health of the mind. The cause of foggy thinking, as I have discovered for myself, is so often found in cellular health.

It took, I believe, many years for my cellular health to return, and even longer for that health to radiate throughout my whole person. And of course I helped this process in many different ways on many different levels, but addressing the root is vital to whole person healing.

Cellular health = Emotional health = Mental health = Spiritual health

When the energy of the cells is flowing and they are absorbing and eliminating efficiently and happily, this energy is passed to every organ of the body, and when every organ of the body is energised and moving minerals, vitamins, hormones and blood at its greatest potential it simply is not rocket-science to imagine that this is going to emanate to the highest vibrational levels of being, the mind and the spirit. The cells are a microcosm of you. They want the same things you do, yet do not have the same power of choice as you. They need great quality oxygen, water, nutrients, and vitamins. But they also need sleep, love, respect, good elimination pathways and a healthy environment to exist and co-exist in. If we only understood and paid attention to the needs and welfare of our cells we would improve our health by extraordinary amounts.

My health now is powerful and strong, yet fluid and relaxed. The body is supple but the core health is strong. My muscle tone is good, and skin is healthy and blemish free. Because my default lifestyle is healthy, supported by regular exercise and vibrant organic (mostly) raw fruits and vegetables, there is never much build up of toxicity. I have certain protocols I use to cleanse toxins built up from the environment, and periodically I address the organs and other needs of my body (liver cleanse for example). But more than that, the life I live is one of the deepest commitment to truth and love. My marriage totally supports this which means life is lived consciously and lovingly, and nothing is allowed to sink into the dark recesses to fester and stagnate or build up an emotional charge. I attend thoroughly to my health on all levels. And this does not in any way mean a tightness or fanatical ruthlessness. It is born out of love and joy. I know that when I am relaxed and well, life flows through me, my creativity flourishes, my power emanates, people are touched by it, I fulfil some purpose in the world and add to the collective wave of transformation.

Completion

As my personal story nears completion and we move on to Part Two of the book and what insights I have gathered that might be useful, I want to talk about a couple of points that contradict popular thinking.

The first is, did I actually have a 'disease'? And the second is, the turning of what appeared to be a great burden in my life to my greatest blessing.

Did I actually have a 'disease'?

Inside this one simple question hides an entire paradigm of thought and belief. We have been trained and conditioned to believe, almost mindlessly without question, that disease is real. It arrives mysteriously, the cause of ostly beyond our understanding and the cure unlikely but remotely possible.

Everyone believes in disease. I have read many books by healers, naturopaths and raw food gurus and the consensus among them is that the idea of disease is a misnomer and a 'red herring.' Put simply, their view is that the body is a highly effective self-organising and self-healing organism composed of a hundred trillion cells all working for the survival and benefit of the whole. So called 'disease' is no more than the body working to isolate or remove impurities and foreign invaders. The function of healing should be to support this process holistically and not to 'treat' it symptomatically. Treating the symptoms of the so-called disease without uncovering and addressing the root cause cannot and will not ever result in the long term healing of the patient.

Personally speaking, I actually do not believe I ever had anything called ulcerative colitis. I do believe I had ulceration of the colon but I believe everything that happened was an intelligent attempt by the body to heal itself. I believe I had a blocked colon, cellular 'constipation' and lymphatic congestion. I also had massive heat in my body from accumulation of foreign bodies (toxins) built up over the years. Although my body, particularly my liver, had succeeded in containing and mitigating these pathogens over the years, it caused wear and tear and great attrition. After my Panchakarma experience the body jumped into super cleansing mode, probably too fast for my system to handle, and the effect was *'colitis-like symptoms.'*

And if I were to have accepted the diagnosis on face value and followed the medication protocol I would have become another statistic of colitis sufferers treated by generic medication for a generic condition with generic symptoms.

But, and this is the point, *we are not generic beings.* We are highly individualised persons with utterly different lives and stories. We have not eaten the same diet, we have not thought the same thoughts or felt the same feelings. Our genetic history is different. What creates the conditions for colitis like symptoms in one person is completely different in another person. These bodily effects need to be treated on an individualised and holistic basis for healing to take place. Treating these conditions generically will never bring healing.

And maybe you will say, "Well it doesn't matter whether we call it disease or not." But actually it does. Our beliefs about whether healing is possible or not possible are connected to what we believe about disease and what we believe is possible. If we believe disease has arrived mysteriously because of a virus, germs or hereditary, that it has very little to do with the lifestyle choices we have made and even less to do with our emotions, and we believe, as I was told, that it is not possible to heal this 'disease,' the chances are we are never going to either try or succeed.

I have seen that those people who really believe they have contracted a disease as if a magic spell has been cast upon them fail to take enough responsibility for the creation or healing of their illness. They rarely heal.

If my story has any power, it is because I chose not to believe I had a disease and not to believe I could not 'cure' it. I gave these terms little attention and did not think in 'medical speak.' I just walked my own path and trusted more and more and left the rest in the hands of the divine. It has been a profound teaching.

Therapies I Have Used

This list might be of some use to you. As you can see I have done many things in my life to heal. Some of them are very powerful. All these happened at the right time for me and I highly recommend all of them.

- Body-Work for emotional release
- Training in Ayurvedic massage
- Training as a wellness coach
- 3 Panchakarmas in Mumbai, India
- Primal Therapy at Miasto Osho Centre, Italy
- Rebirthing sessions (many)
- Enlightenment Intensive
- 1-year Shamanic Contemplation Training with Spirit Horse Nomadic Circle (Wales)
- Vision quest, mountain top vigil, cave vigil, sweat lodge, fire ceremonies

- Family Constellation Work, both participating and running programs
- Psychosynthesis
- Mens Warrior Training
- Tantra Training
- Osho Meditations (Dynamic, Kundalini)
- Vipassana Training x 2
- Chi Kung, Yoga, Tai Chi
- Exercise - running, interval training, strength training, cycling, swimming
- Rebounding
- Meditation
- Visualisations and Affirmations
- Self-inquiry
- Fasting

PART TWO

THE POWER TO CHANGE

INTRODUCTION

In Part One of this book I related my story. Now I'm going to talk to you about what I learned along the way that might be useful. It has been a long and, at times, tough journey. I have had to dig deep, persist and trust. I have had to find new inner resources. I have had to learn new information. Sometimes I feel like a private investigator! In short, I have had to totally recreate myself and become my own healer. I had to strip away everything that was false in order to let the light shine through. It has been a warrior's journey.

Now that I understand so much better the journey and all it involves, I feel I may have something to offer those who may find themselves in a similar situation.

I don't know what will heal you, what remedies, what particular foods, exactly what protocol you should use. But I do know that pretty much anything is possible. I know how things link up, I understand the interconnectedness between things. I know the areas it might be worth focusing on when dealing with illness. I understand the momentum of the wave of healing and how it rises and falls. And I know how to inspire others to pick

on and join the race. That is what Part Two is
You need energy to change. You need commit-
guts to take the healing path. Any path that
steers away from the conventional is arduous because it
means you have to actively get involved. We are so used
to handing over our power and authority to experts that,
when it comes to our health, we get terrified of the alternatives. And the corporations prey on our fear.

Consider, for one moment, how many times when you were very young, you visited the doctor or were told you may visit the doctor. Every little cough, fever and cut had the potential to deliver us to the doctor's surgery. And of course our vaccinations were performed by the doctor. The 'doctor' plays an integral part in the life of a developing family. And this is as it should be when the doctor is wise, kindly, independent of thought, and has the best interests of the community at heart. The image of the gentle and caring family doctor is persistent.

But when we get older and develop chronic conditions and our doctors no longer have time for us and are under such pressure to distribute the latest medication that they pay little attention to so called alternative healing methods, then what options are we left with? And doctors actually know nothing about diet or chronic conditions. Suppose you actively want to experiment with alternatives? 90% of doctors and other professionals will attempt to dissuade you, citing unproven dangers and hearsay. It is all geared towards the mainstream, and whilst that is fine for many people, it is not fine for everyone. 'Doctor' is firmly embedded in our consciousness and it is very hard to break this automatic response mechanism that makes us reach out to him (or her). And of course, sometimes it is vital we go to the doctor. But we need to develop much more discernment over when those times are.

This book is for those who want to seek other possibilities. You may have to walk alone. But there are thousands, probably millions of other people, also walking alone.

It is vital that we as individuals wake up and play our part in the conscious change in the world. Our health is not separate from that. It is crucial.

And the most powerful thing about illness is its capacity to shake us up and wake us up.

Of course it feels frightening, but that's the price of liberation. Illness presents us with an option of taking an active part in the experience of our lives, looking at what might have contributed to our ill health and changing it, or handing over all our power to professionals and abdicating responsibility, as though our current predicament has nothing to do with us. And mostly it is a blend of both using professional knowledge and our own inner guidance. But it is your life, and you must become the master of your destiny.

I am amazed by how easily so many people give up their own power just to stay within the confines of their own beliefs. It's called *'the comfort zone.'* It's not that comfortable and it doesn't lead to transformation or healing.

Those who heal, every one of them, have had to step out of their comfort zone. They have all had to change something. And some people just cannot do it. The older you are the more difficult it tends to be. My own father couldn't do it, it just wasn't available for him as an idea or a concept or a possibility. And that is ok as well.

But for you it may be possible, as it was for me. This book is for you.

I am going to offer you the lessons I have learned on my journey of healing. Some are spiritual, some are physical, and some emotional. I will talk about detoxification, and I will talk about food. The point of this book is to inspire you to look into all this for yourself. It is, if anything, motivational. And forgive me if I miss anything out. The path of life is one of mystery. I myself have often felt fated to be doing this. I never intended to be writing about health, well-being or transformation. I was (and still am) a musician who became very ill. But life made me pay attention, it drew me up close and whispered in my ear with such tenderness I had to listen. And in listening my heart broke at my own story, my own sadness, anger and pain. And I understood the purpose of my life was to heal through love, compassion, gratitude and forgiveness. I was compelled by my own soul to walk the path, and I walked and walked. Eventually something changed within, a kind of maturation. Maybe it is a sort of wisdom. I definitely know myself more than I ever did, and I love myself unconditionally.

And once I reached a certain point it became absolutely obvious that I was going to share this with other people. It was a choiceless choice. So here I am, both compelled and delighted to offer you something that may encourage your healing, your transformation, and your heart opening. May the force of love be with you!

From Burden to Blessing

As I have emerged from my darkest periods when I really did feel very burdened by a massive wound I thought I would never recover from, I have slowly started to reframe the entire experience and put it into the context of my life. And when I look at it in this light I see that, far from it being the worst thing that could have happened to me, it is the best thing.

It has not been a burden but a blessing.

It has transformed every single aspect of my being. Physically, I am stronger and healthier now than ever. Illness forced me to look at everything I ate and drank, forced me to face all my addictive tendencies and become informed and intelligent about what heals the body and what harms it. And it keeps me reminded of this each and every day. Indulgence is a thing of the past for me. Emotionally, I had to turn and face all my demons, all the unloved parts of myself. I unlocked them from my suffering body and released them from my bag of woes. From being a man who could barely even say the word love I wrote and released an album called 'Unconditional Love.' I talk about love, I sing about love and I am unafraid of love. Mentally, I had to meet my conditioned self with all its inherited beliefs and values. That was a challenge, and sometimes it still is. Conditioning is deeply embedded and very hard to disentangle. Spiritually, I was invited to look at my relationship with God, the universe, and divine intelligence.

As each area of my life has healed at deeper and ever more subtle levels, a growing grace and gratitude has come upon me and I have realised that it was my distorted perception that saw what was happening to me as a burden, but life is always an invitation to awaken and go deeper, and gradually this perception shifted and now it appears as such a wonderful opportunity to grow. I now see all experiences in life as opportunities and invitations to know myself deeper and more wisely.

I truly see the phrases 'Know Thyself' and 'Heal Thyself' everywhere in daily life.

SHORT ESSAY ON SYMPTOMS

Consider this scenario … You have a car and the warning light on the dashboard keeps coming on, causing you some concern. You take the car to a mechanic, he takes the car into the rear of the garage, snips the wire that connects to the light and returns the car to you and says, 'the problem is solved.' And off you go about your daily business.

How long before the car breaks down?

What I'm describing is a trip to the doctor for many people experiencing the things we call symptoms.

The doctor is the mechanic.

The pharmaceuticals are the wire cutters.

Your body is the engine that continues to try and send the warning signals to you, the driver, but now has to try and find another route.

Put bluntly, you will still have the cause of the symptoms but no symptoms. *Am I the only one to think that is crazy?*

Let us talk about symptom suppression. Sometimes it works, sometimes it helps buy some time while another intervention takes place. Believe me, I am not anti medication. If it truly works, I am absolutely in favour. But I need to see that it really works and enables healing, proper healing of cells, tissues and organs. I need to see that medication is not just putting the problem off until some point in the future, like sticking our head in the sand. I really need to know that or I just cannot see the point in doing it. I would rather deal with a serious problem now than a hopeless situation later on. I don't just want to buy time. If illness comes along I intend to listen to what it has to say and endeavour to transform the situation and create better health.

I see the same thing in every health centre, every ward in every hospital and every surgery, people trying to cope with chronic illness but looking for the easiest way without having to make any changes in their lives. That is neither possible nor reasonable. It is not going to happen. And the whole idea of symptom suppression feeds on this.

If you remember from my story, I decided right from the start that I would not take drugs for my dis-ease. I really believe that decision was crucial. You see my body only had to focus on the cause of the inflammation. It did not have to also deal with the effect of the medication. My liver was overloaded enough with the toxic burden it already had. If I added the 'side-effects' of the meds it might have been too much. Because this is the truth: medication is not natural, it is synthetic, which means it is alien to the body. For all the benefit it gives, and obviously it gives benefit, it puts a huge burden on the body to deal with the toxic side effects. It is a balancing act. I was not prepared to go down that route.

My symptoms were strong and extremely worrying. They were not extreme enough to take me to hospital. An acute life-threatening experience has to be dealt with, there is no question. I am not a fool arguing naively against all medication. I am a mature adult with many years personal experience of symptoms and dis-ease and I have arrived at a place where I am not at all convinced by this current attitude of 'throw drugs at the problem and get them back to work.' It is insane and either the method of ignorance or evil, probably both.

I have also benefitted from medication. Antibiotics worked for me when nothing else did, and painkillers have resolved an extreme headache when I was desperate. But I always sought to resolve the root cause. After antibiotics I always took probiotics and ate fermented foods, and looked into why I needed to take them in the first place. I didn't rest until I found an understanding and then I took action, radical and dramatic action. If I had medicated all the times the doctors wanted me to I would be a walking medicine cabinet. They have tried to diagnose me with Raynaud's condition, scleroderma, and Hashimoto's disease as well as the inflammatory bowel disease. I did not buy any of it and used all my powers to look deeper and deeper within and treated the root cause. And then the symptoms began to disappear.

That's what happens. Symptoms disappear when the root cause is healed. But it is tough to swim against the tide of everyone else's opinion, and the backing of this medical science stuff. Because mad though it may sound, we live in a world where we actually all believe that if you get rid of the symptoms, by whatever means, then you have got rid of the problem! I mean I am still shocked even as I write that.

Symptoms are indicators, they are, in fact, possibly one of the best friends you can have. Symptoms are the body's intelligent way of saying, 'look here, take notice of this, it needs your attention.' It is impossible for us to be on track all the time, we are human beings in organic bodies walking through the world. Things are going to happen inside us. We have massive cell die-off all the time, illness arises, there are innate weaknesses in bodies, which means we need to know what is happening and takes steps to bring harmony inside. That's what symptoms are about. Supreme intelligence has given us this gift. If we get swelling, head pain, inflammation, back pain, gut pain, or spots, it is an indication of some imbalance happening inside us. The body is trying to remove the issue. We need to take measures to address the situation. Most of the time medication will not be the answer. This means you are going to have to look elsewhere if you are serious about healing.

Healing is very possible if you are serious enough about taking the appropriate steps towards it, not halfway steps and not compromised steps.

Drive your car consciously. If the red warning light comes on make sure that if and when you go to the mechanic doctor you ask 'What do you think is causing this red light?' See what answer you get. Before he snips the wire to the light try and find out what caused it to light up. Don't just keep driving the car regardless, the consequences could be serious. And if the doctor can't answer (and my bet is that he/she can't) then find someone who can. Try the natural and 'alternative' medicines. Try Chinese or Ayurvedic medicine. Try a Naturopath or Acupuncturist, you will be surprised to find that symptoms can be easy to read. Then, and only then, you can take action to mediate the symptoms.

ILLNESS IS AN OPPORTUNITY

When illness knocks at your door

When illness knocks at your door
Let it in, it may be a friend
Or a guide sent by the Divine
To remind you of something
Lost in time.
Sit down and listen to their tale,
They may open a window
To your soul
Or hold up a mirror and show you a picture
Of yourself
You have never seen before.
Don't shut them out on that cold night
Don't leave them alone to weep their tears of sorrow.
Bring them in and show them the warmth of your love
Hold them with your charity
And they will reveal deep truths
And hidden worlds,
And secrets you have forgotten.

> *'Every situation, properly perceived, becomes an opportunity to heal'* - Course in Miracles

Of course it is natural that if illness arrives in your life you are not going to jump with joy. It is very hard to even accept it, particularly if it is serious, painful or life threatening, let alone welcome it. This, I am acutely aware, is a very delicate subject. It is easy, once we have healed or are no longer in pain, to say let illness be an opportunity to heal some part of yourself, but it is indeed very tough *at the time.* However, what I am going to say in this chapter could be so very useful to you or to someone you love that it may help support you through the difficult times.

It is all about how we respond to situations.

If you are experiencing illness, particularly if it is one of the 'chronic conditions,' which means it is deeply embedded and is linked to lifestyle choices, you are going to have to create a lot of energy to heal. This energy needs to be as positive as possible. And that means your attitude at the time is crucial to healing. That is the context of this chapter. It's not easy, and there are always times when it is impossible to view illness as an opportunity to grow, like during crisis or intense pain, but when these times fade we can return to a commitment to our healing.

One of the reasons I have been so successful in healing my inflammatory bowel disease and going from such a state of toxic overload to my current state of health is that I seized the opportunity that my illness offered me. And that meant I took radical action. It was not always easy but I am tenacious and committed, and even during the negative days when I felt all was lost and I would be sick forever and life was over, I persisted and didn't 'cave in.'

Remember, becoming ill brings you to a knife-edge in your life. You become the tightrope walker over the great ravine. When the body screams at you 'You have to do something different, you have to take notice here because I am in system collapse,' then things have reached the danger zone. In order to get to some state of health and wellness, you cannot just go backwards to the way things were. You can't just cement over the cracks and carry on as normal. You may well find yourself, to continue the analogy, having to take down the whole wall, clean the entire place and rebuild it with new plaster and paint.

And that is where you see the opportunity.

It is the chance to transform the room, with fresh plaster, a new lick of paint, and a massive clear up. The room would be like a new room. Will it require a lot of work? Yes. Is there a lot of preparation work involved? Yes. Do you have to commit to the whole journey? Yes. Is it really worth it? Yes Yes Yes. There is a Samurai Warrior's Creed written anonymously in the 14th Century. Among it's amazing words I found this:

'I have no design: I make seizing opportunity by the forelock my design.'

This is what I am pointing to, the power to seize this experience as an opportunity to look within, to take stock of oneself and to make important decisions to change those things that have contributed to illness, or just those things that don't work in your life. It is the opportunity, in fact it is the grandest opportunity, to heal your life, to transform any negativity, to reach a new understanding, to heal your broken heart, to change lifestyle habits, relationships, toxic patterns. It is the opportunity to inhabit your body fully, and let go of stuck emotions from the past. It is the opportunity to remember what is truly important in life and to live from that place. And it is an opportunity to remember your sacredness and spirituality.

It is very rare in our busy lives that we get the chance to reflect and reconsider, some never do it to the day they die, and here comes life with this window of opportunity.

In fact, if you look at this very closely, it is not 'life' that has come along and offered you this opportunity. It is, in fact, you. Your actions, your thoughts, your beliefs, your diet choices, your lifestyle habits, your relationships, your connection with your spirit, maybe even your karma, all these have conspired to bring you to this place. The least you can do is honour yourself!

The majority of people live on the surface of their lives. Life, when truly contemplated, has such depth and grandeur to it, like a deep ocean, and yet most of the time we are as the waves on the surface, preoccupied with the business of being a wave and forgetful of the deep ocean beneath us. We are conditioned and trained to conform to the values and beliefs of the society we live in.

And as such we gather up many subconscious expectations about our lives. And illness doesn't belong in those expectations. If illness arrives on our doorstep it confounds us and punches a hole in those expectations. It is a big confrontation.

So we all agree it is the worst thing that could possibly happen, and if only you could get rid of it as fast as possible and return to 'normal' life then everything will be ok again. Suggesting that illness is an opportunity for transformation, when viewed in this context, sounds ludicrous and almost insane. But we are not born to be so disconnected from our true self, we are not designed to carry so much unresolved emotion, and we are not capable of maintaining health if we eat toxic foods.

This modern disconnected lifestyle is killing us.

We maintain it by consensus, and if some poor soul gets sick it strikes fear into the heart of everyone. That fear is both a real concern on a genuine human level for that person, but also a fear that something is rocking the boat, triggering deeper issues that live in everyone. Those issues are the things we avoid in life, the deepest of questions. Who am I? What happens when I die? What is the meaning of this life? Am I happy? What is my true purpose? What is love?

It is fear that prevents us from embracing illness. This fear is both personal and collective. It is very real. I am certainly not saying the fear is wrong, far from it. *I am saying that the fear is right!* Denying it, pushing it away, pretending it is not there, covering it up with denial, maintaining a 'stiff upper lip,' hoping it will go away, these are powerful obstacles to embracing our illness and the healing journey.

And to compound the problem, the conventional medical model is driven by this fear. It wants to get you out as quickly as possible, get you on your feet and work/home with little fuss. Or it wants you on medication for the rest of your life.

As you can probably imagine, if someone then embraces their illness as an opportunity for transformation, not only is it going to challenge them, it is also going to challenge their family, friends, work colleagues and the professionals they consult. It is a big deal. But if you are called to the healing path, this is the deal. You may have to make some tough decisions that to others will look crazy, and may even make you feel crazy. If you want to transform, heal, let go, forgive, and find something deeper, this is part of the trip.

Ending the War with Illness

Illness does not arrive in our life as a gift or an opportunity. It arrives, generally speaking, as an unwelcome problem. It is uninvited. It is going to get in the way and cause a lot of trouble. It is, in fact, a curse. At least that is the conventional view of it. And like all things that are unwelcome in our society we have only one approach we can take.

We declare war on it.

We declare war on the very thing that is trying to tell us something. We simply have no conception that our body might be trying to tell us something about ourselves, so we see it as the enemy, something we have to get rid off as soon as possible. Think of the endless 'war on cancer.' Has it done any good?

It is going to involve a conscious decision on your part to start viewing it in a different way. That conscious decision is to step away from the declaration of war and start making peace with illness. You do this by allowing it in. What I mean by allowing it in is that you start working with it, not against it. There is a big difference. And what I'm talking about is not resignation to having illness, let's just clear that up. I have seen so many ill people accept their fate with the air of doomed resignation, as though they are utterly powerless in the face of it.

Opening to illness and allowing it to inform and teach us says, '*I am available and open, show me what I need to change, show me how I can transform. I'm scared but I am still going to stay open.*' Resigning to illness has a very different voice, it says, '*I give up, I am resigned to my fate. There is no point in trying to do anything. I'm so scared I'm not going to listen.*'

Which voice would you listen to?

Disengagement?

Don't get the idea that what I'm saying is that you passively disengage from your illness, accept it and not do anything. That could not be further from the truth. I moved heaven and earth to heal myself. I still do. I take massive action. It is the only way to heal. No one wants to be ill, and everyone, including me, wants to get it resolved as soon as possible. We all want health. But war is not the answer to anything, inside the body or outside it. The body is a highly intelligent act of creation evolved over millions of years. It has an intelligence we ignore and know very little about.

The body breaks down for a reason. Sometimes it is a technical problem, or a genetic malfunction, or an attack from outside, but not often. The vast majority of illnesses and diseases are connected to and caused by lifestyle choices. That means, in a nutshell, that illness is connected to our behaviour, and our behaviour is connected to our beliefs. So if an illness, particularly a chronic illness, shows up in our lives, it has something very important to tell us about our behaviour and our beliefs. Beliefs drive behaviour.

The wise listen. The foolish ignore.

Everything happens for a reason

The guiding principle of my life, my healing and even my coaching, is that everything happens for a reason. We may not always know what that reason is and sometimes it eludes us for years, but there is a deeper intelligence at work that guides everything. As consciousness, or even as a soul incarnated on earth, you are here to learn and evolve. You can only do this by having experiences and then reflecting and learning from them.

And really, who are we to judge whether something is good or bad, right or wrong? Who are we to say this should happen and this shouldn't happen?

I am reminded of the great teacher Byron Katie who in her powerful 'The Work' brings people out of their judgement to a place of deeper surrender and love. She would ask of someone who is ill, 'Can you know definitely, absolutely, that you shouldn't be ill right now?' and the answer is always no.

So maybe it is ok that you are ill. Maybe it's exactly the right thing for you right now. Maybe it is indeed the greatest opportunity you have had so far in your life to become more of yourself. You might become more open, wiser, deeper, lighter, more joyous, even healthier! You might find new purpose and meaning. You might find the authentic spiritual connection that every human being yearns for. You might start doing all the creative things you ever wanted to do but never found the time for. This opportunity could change everything. It all depends on how you respond.

HEALING THE EMOTIONAL ROOTS OF ILLNESS

'Your task is to let go of something painful to receive something pleasurable.'

A conversation about the connection between emotions, illness and healing is worthy of a book in itself. Some people even postulate that if we could heal our toxic buried emotions we would manifest amazing health simply by the release of energy. You certainly cannot achieve excellent whole person health without balanced and flowing emotions. And of course they don't always have to be joyful. They just have to be authentically you. Energy is intended to flow from the highest realms into the lowest realms and be released to flow back again. That means energy flows from what we call spirit down into the human vehicle, we 'feel' our experiences and call them joy, shame, anger etc, based on our previous experience, and some of these 'feelings,' the ones we cannot allow to flow through, get lodged in the body as trapped energy. Energy must circulate. Trapped energy becomes stagnant or toxic in the body. And this is the root cause of many diseases. Certain emotions relate to certain bodily areas because the body is a sophisticated and super intelligent reflection of us, our mind, our thoughts and our spirit. The medical view of the body is sadly lacking in its understanding of this and society suffers as a result.

We need to develop a much more intuitive and holistic approach to illness that truly recognises the intertwined relationship between body, emotion, mind and spirit. Treating illness on purely the physical level is a sad reflection of the naivety of our society.

We cannot say where the body finishes and emotions start. They are the same thing. Emotion is expressed through the body. Emotion is energy in motion in the body.

When this energy, what we call emotion, is no longer in motion, it will, over time, begin to express itself in the body as 'symptoms.' These symptoms are designed to remind us to release the energy by resolving whatever caused it to stagnate in the first place. It's a highly intelligent feedback system.

Most of us who have become chronically ill need to let go of something we have been carrying a long time. It is usually some toxic emotion, or the lack of self love. There is always something fundamental at the root of illness. When we move away from love, the guiding force of the universe, we are already ill in our being. It is inevitable this will manifest in our bodies.

Look at my story and tell me what created my illness, emotions or lifestyle?

It is impossible to separate these things out. Emotions are connected to beliefs, which are created by our experiences. Our beliefs dictate our habits, our relationships, and the choices we make each and every day, over and over again. So to heal our lives, ill or not, at some point we must engage with our core beliefs.

Before we dive in a little deeper to the mystery of emotions and illness, I want to make it clear. Toxic emotions kill people. We see this all the time in suicide. We see it in murder and in things like eating disorders. These are the more dramatic views we have, but strangely when it come to chronic illness that affects millions of people we tend not, as a society, to understand the connection. It's a convenient blind spot.

I have experienced directly and powerfully how old traumas undigested and unreleased live in the body. I was shocked by the power of this revelation. And they don't just live passively, they live chronically, festering and gathering more toxicity towards them.

I lived as though I was in a prison, walled in and unable to access my true power or joy or love. My creativity was an expression of pain, like so many artists. I wore a mask of happiness and I became an excellent actor playing the part of Kavi in my life. But there was no fulfilment, no inner peace, and no real health. I had a reputation for many years as being impossible to hug. I could barely say the word love even though I was in a committed relationship. The suppression of my anger and fear had driven me almost mad over the years and led me to massive drug abuse and dependence on alcohol. It took years of commitment and diving in to my pain for me to release the trauma and heal the wounds. I believe now that it is possible to shorten the journey with awareness and a more focused approach, and that is why I am writing this book.

Unravelling emotions

The purpose of life is love. That doesn't mean just loving someone, it means love at the core level of being. It means *being love*, giving unconditional love and receiving unconditional love. The vibrational power of love in its true form is extraordinary. It touches everyone. Consider the power of Jesus to heal and transform others. That is the power of love. But most of us never get to touch this power ever in our lives. We are so wounded and diminished over the generations that we live as though we know what love is, yet we are far away from it, living as shadows of love. We are shadows.

> *The potential power of illness gives us the opportunity to return to this love, to unlock the doors and remove all the blocks and to become the embodiment of this unconditionality. Healing is the path of returning to the love we came from.*

The vulnerability with which we enter the world as a baby leaves us at the mercy of our parents or carers. Depending on their maturity, karma, balance, love, and of course their own history, our experience and learning about ourselves and the world becomes defined by them.

For some born to loving parents this is extremely nourishing and supporting. But for others it is not always an easy ride. Some endure horror and carry the scars for life. But everyone is impacted by their childhood.

And childhood is where we learn what to do with our emotions. We learn which ones 'are allowed,' which ones leave us feeling unloved and which ones get us what we want. It is all about love, getting love.

Our hearts so easily become walled in and protected as love is bartered, battered, manipulated and smashed. Its part of growing up. If I paint a bleak picture it is to make the point, it's not to blame anyone, for everyone has their own story of pain and ultimately in forgiveness there is no one to blame. I am talking about what may need to be healed if there is illness, although I have to add I have never met anyone, sick or well, who could not benefit from healing their emotions.

These are the things we learn when we are very young. There are also, of course, experiences we have during our entire youth that contribute to our emotional health. Consider my childhood. As far as I know, for the first ten years it was nourishing. I was innocent of the trauma of the world and lived as a child of the 60s, free and careless, with two loving parents who I thought of as Gods and who could do no wrong. I ran in the fields, played outdoors all the time and loved life with such an excitement it was incredible. And then from age ten or so, my family life imploded like a chronic illness, and I was torn apart until at sixteen I was jettisoned out into the world, alone and ill equipped to know what to do.

Everyone who carries illness has to heal something from their youth. There is always some part of them that has withdrawn from love, or felt unloved, rejected or abandoned. Find it, love it and heal it. That is the task of the modern health warrior.

What are the benefits of this painful task?

It can be painful stirring up old memories. It takes strength, courage and vulnerability. But these are the tools of the warrior of the heart.

In my experience I have noticed this. That it is the fear of these emotions that actually hold us back from dealing with them, not the emotions themselves. Fear is the big thing and its fear that keeps us walled in. When we really meet fear and allow it, breathe with it, it actually dissolves, and what lies behind it is love and vulnerability.

Fear is the mask that shields wounded love.

Love is open and vulnerable. As a child or youth it is so easy to retract and protect the vulnerable and open heart, but it doesn't lead to a full and joyous life.

You let go of the pain to receive the pleasure of life.

- She goes consciously into the shadows to tackle the dragons and demons of the past, knowing she will fly into freedom when they are slayed.

- He weeps for the pain he felt, he rages at his memories, knowing the peace that is underneath.
- She releases herself from the bondage of guilt and shame, knowing it no longer serves her.
- He forgives his parents, carers and abusers because holding onto the pain only hurts him and creates illness and unhappiness.
- She actively chooses joy, love, gratitude, compassion and freedom.

The benefits, direct and indirect, of releasing old emotions can be:

- A profound release of positive energy.
- An ability to flow with life more easily.
- More connection and depth in all relationships.
- A deeper sense of inner peace and calm.
- Greater sense of purpose.
- A new meaning to life.
- Joy.

The physical effects can be:

- Healthy impact on digestion and elimination.
- Reduction of stress in body.
- Immune system benefits.
- Adrenal system benefits.

- More energy.
- Better absorption.
- Heart health and blood pressure improvements.
- Greater clarity of mind.

There are thousands of fringe benefits that you won't see. Everything is connected to everything else, so no matter where you take action, it is going to change things.

Healed emotions create more healthy choices. We are no longer victims of our choices, driven by the need to get love or avoid pain, but a master of them.

The greatest benefit of healing emotions, the one thing I want to convey more than anything else, is the sense of freedom this delivers into our lives. I cannot begin to describe how this has improved the quality and depth of every aspect of my existence, from my food choices, to my creativity and to my relationships.

I am as a free man, and it is such a liberation.

Moving through life burdened and shackled by the past is half a life. Letting it all go and coming into the present moment unshackled and unchained is joy itself. Consciousness was not meant to be tied down by the past, we owe it to ourselves to drop the baggage and step forward into this freedom. We are always being invited to let go and live now.

How to release old toxic emotions?

As I have said before, my book is primarily aimed at the *why* not the *how*. We are each guided in our unique directions. No two journeys are the same, and what worked for me may not work for you. It is all about making the journey, walking the path and taking the action guided by your intuition, those professionals you are drawn to and a certain amount of investigation. My journey was, and still is, quite incredible in the twists and turns it has taken, being led here and there to this person and that modality, a few blind alleys but always moving and changing. So it is for you.

All it really requires is willingness.

Sure, there are some modalities I will list, but there is also a powerful yet subtle way you can act that involves spending no money and seeking no professional help.

It just takes your willingness, in this moment, to meet any emotion as it arises and to not deflect or avoid it at all. Just being with it, no story or excuse, not even a label that calls it anger or shame. Just the energy as it arises in your body consciousness. Some of the more dramatic emotions that lodge in the body need help to cathart and release. But others simply need to be allowed and embraced, held and loved as a mother holds a crying child. Nothing needs to be done. And in difficult moments of feeling 'triggered' when you might be reaching for some comforting food, or drink, or cigarette, or the tv, choose not to.

Take that one moment and hit the pause button. Breathe. Consciously sit and ask, 'what am I experiencing right now?' Allow memories, feelings, sensations, to rise up. Don't even name them, and don't even try to heal them. In truth we do not heal them, we just allow them to un-stick and go their own way. If tears come, let them, if anger comes, let it, and if fear arises, be ok with it. Feel it but don't shrink from it. Just sitting and allowing these feelings and sensations and emotions to rise creates space and moves energy. And this is the point. What rises also falls. We are afraid of demons, but mostly what we are afraid of is the fear itself.

Our pushing away of these emotions, our fear that they will crush us, is what has given them power over us. But it is not the truth. Only fear has power over us. So allow them, let them in and through, even if it feels as though your heart will break. It won't. It can't. This is the power of Present Moment Awareness. It can only break open.

I am a great believer that the way to healing is by allowing the wall that protects the heart to come down and crumble to dust. It is a great metaphor and I use it all the time. The protection we thought the wall gave us is an illusion. It keeps us trapped. Allowing your heart to break open allows the river of love to flow. That river of love is the healing balm of life. When the river of love is truly flowing, it no longer matters what happens to the physical body. If it heals there is love. If it dies there is love. It is that powerful.

Do not be scared of opening your heart, be scared of not opening your heart.

Other modalities for healing trauma and toxic emotions:

Breath-work (Rebirthing) – This is an extremely powerful process. Through the power of the breath in a session with a therapist you will, over a period of time, dislodge those emotions in your body. Breath is the most powerful tool. I absolutely recommend this for anyone, regardless of whether they are ill or not. I have done scores of breath-work sessions and I can personally testify to their efficacy.

Body-work – Designed specifically for the purpose of releasing stuck emotion in the body, there are many variations from Reichian body work to the Feldenkrais technique, and scores of others. Absolutely guaranteed to help you.

Primal Therapy – As powerful as it gets. We devoted two weeks to the process of stirring things up, letting them out, inner child work, and all held in the bowl of meditation. (This was at one of Osho's Centres in Italy)

Family Constellation – Even though it is not a 'cathartic' technique there is a power of healing in this extraordinary experience that shifts energy in a (sometimes) mysterious way.

Psychosynthesis – Put simply this therapy focuses on our 'sub-personalities,' the often wounded parts of us that we carry unconsciously around and who only make their presence felt when we are 'triggered' by some event or memory. This therapy is a powerful healing tool that brings awareness and integration of our fragmented parts. Once again I can vouch for the power of this therapy, it arrived in my life at exactly the right time and opened my eyes and my heart to myself on a deep and profound level.

CELLULAR INTELLIGENCE

"You may consider yourself an individual... but you are in truth a cooperative community of approximately fifty-trillion single-celled citizens." - **Bruce Lipton**

There is an intelligence inside you that has an awareness that matches and even surpasses yours. It is a collective consciousness, a symbiotic community that has developed over millennia. In many ways this vast community is more advanced than our own national and international societies. They work together, getting individual needs met and also contributing to the whole in a selfless way. They are organised and function at an extraordinary level of cooperation. When the entire community is working at its optimum and in a state of harmony guess what happens? You feel great! You are healthy, vibrant and balanced.

This vast community is your cellular world. It is the unseen but very real world that is you. But here is the rub. This cellular community is as dependent on you as you are on it. It is an incredibly symbiotic relationship. If you care (consciously) for it by feeding it the right foods, giving it good water, loving it and giving it positive thoughts, it will reward you by giving you energy, creativity, clarity and a deep sense of goodness and love.

It is probably not too crazy to suppose that dis-ease is nothing more than a breakdown in the relationship between us and our cells. And if you are ill or you want to take your health, even your life in general, to a new level then taking a good look at your cellular health is an excellent place to start. As you will see, the relationship you have with your cells on the physical, emotional, mental and energetic levels is one that can define everything about how healthy, sick, energetic, creative and contented you are. We take them for granted. We barely think about them. We have a huge disconnect about them, even the doctors and medical world are not going to mention them ever in your consultation.

But if you go to some more advanced naturopaths and alternative healers, your cells are the only thing they are going to talk about.

You have approximately fifty-trillion, some say even a hundred-trillion, cells in your body. Your body is cells, cells and fluid. That's all it is, cells and fluid. Skin cells, blood cells, brain cells, tissue cells, etc.

If something is physically wrong with you, it is wrong with your cells. Illness is cellular malfunction. No matter what dis-ease it may be called, at its root it is cellular malfunction. Cells need nourishment to function. Deprived of nourishment they suffer, as we do. What nourishment do they need? Oxygen, water, amino acids, glucose, essential fatty acids, minerals and vitamins. They also need to eliminate waste matter, the same as us. Millions of cells die each day and they need to be removed from the body. So we need our body fluid moving healthily. That means interstitial fluid and lymph. These cells are uncannily like little people in many ways. They digest food, they assimilate nutrients, and they eliminate waste. If any of these functions are blocked or over burdened there are going to be problems eventually.

The environment the cells live in is very important. It must be a healthy, flowing, alkaline, non-toxic environment to deal with acids and toxins. If the cells cannot eliminate waste it is like your toilet backing up. At some point it is going to overflow and create dis-ease. This is why the alternative health world talks about your lymph system all the time. You have to get this system (the lymph) moving and that requires activity (exercise) and possibly extra nutrition or herbs. It may require sweating or massage. The lymph system has no pump to move the fluid through the body, unlike the venus (blood) system, which means it is prone to getting clogged, particularly with today's acidic mainstream diet.

We are bombarded with toxins. They are in the air we breathe, the water we drink, our food, our household items, our cars and our clothes. They are in our beauty and hair products. Since the beginning of last century the number of chemicals in our environment has steady increased until we are now on absolute overload.

Our bodies, particularly our livers, can cope with a certain amount but the liver of nearly every single person is screaming stop! Toxins, chemicals, synthetic medication, vaccines, additives and scores of other unnatural products, are killing us on the cellular level. If we are struggling on the cellular level then we are struggling on the surface because there is no real difference between the two. They are intrinsically connected.

We are not meant to live, let alone thrive, under this toxic load.

And just when you thought it couldn't get any worse along comes the news about your negative thoughts, toxic emotions and constant stress and anxiety and how they impact your cells.

The structure of each cell in the body gives it an intelligence, a consciousness, an awareness and a sensitivity to its environment. That environment is both its immediate one but also the bigger you. What you think, feel and believe affects your cells as much as what you eat and drink. So finely tuned are your cells that they respond to not only your conscious thoughts and feelings, but also your subconscious beliefs.

The cells in your body know what you are really thinking and what you really believe. You program your cells behaviour with your beliefs.

It has to be this way or we would not have unity between mind and body. Your life might depend on the precision of this relationship. The cells have to be finely tuned to your thoughts and beliefs so that, if you have to run away from danger, they can create the energy instantly to do this. They monitor your mental and emotional activity all the time, moment by moment.

What I'm saying is that if you love yourself unconditionally your cells will respond to it. It bathes them in energetic well-being.

If you hate yourself or if you hate the world, your cells hear this and see no reason to thrive. Its like an emotional acid bath. If you feel life is pointless your cellular world is going to reflect that feeling as depression and fatigue and give you no energy. Your cells don't actually know what is a conscious or unconscious thought, it's the power of the thought they respond to. Consider previous mentions of the placebo and nocebo effect to see the power of the mind on cellular health. It can make us ill or it can make us sick, it is up to us.

And there is another problem. Most people are living lives with the stress button constantly on. Lifestyle habits of the 21st century urban human are fast paced, over toxic, burdened by intense emotions and plagued by negative beliefs and thoughts. If the environmental toxins don't get you, the negative self doubting unloving beliefs will, and they can be even more hazardous!

The western world is in a state of cellular collapse and descent into chronic disease. But we just don't get it and we stumble off to the doctors and treat the symptoms.

I'm sorry to be the bringer of all this bad news, I really am. But it may be true that only by rubbing our noses in it will we really begin to take notice and take action. I get the feeling sometimes that we are all waiting for someone or something else before we jump into full responsibility and action and address some of these major issues. The news is the time is upon us, every one of us, whether we are sick or well, rich or poor, happy or miserable. It all starts with us as individuals.

The good news is, it is not all bad news!

We have been graced with incredible power. That power can heal illness, turn life around and create transformation. The possibilities are there, and all they need is a decision and a willingness to experiment. Think about it. If it is true that our cells will decay, dehydrate and die if they are deprived of the things they need, then surely if we clean up our inner environment, oxygenate, hydrate and nourish our cells, they may well begin to thrive and create health. Maybe our symptoms will disappear.

And if we also transform our self harming and negative thoughts and beliefs, bringing them to the surface and dissolving them, return to self love, gratitude, joy and inner harmony, then surely we can undo dis-ease. We can restore harmony. We can, in effect, become the true benevolent king or queen of our inner kingdom, taking care of each area of our inner world because we love our subjects, our hundred-trillion cells.

This is all about you taking dominion over your life in all its richness and confusion. You are the ruler. You can give that power away, and there are many who will gladly accept power over you, including pharmaceutical and food companies, you can use it negatively against yourself and others and pay the price with physical and emotional problems. Or you can transform yourself into a powerful, wise and kindly ruler, committed to truth, love and freedom. You can commit to nourishing your inner kingdom so that all thrive. You banish negativity and emotional toxicity, you banish self-harm and fear and you transmute dis-ease into opportunity to know yourself deeper and clearer.

Ours is a time of disconnection from ourselves, each other, planet earth and our spiritual source. But there is a profound awakening taking place that seeks to address that very disconnection. It is all about healing disconnection. And disease plays a vital and valuable part of this re-connecting. It offers us an incredible opportunity to re-connect with ourselves and remember who we really are. But only when we step up, take dominion, dive in, take action, rise in conscious awareness and heal. There is not much greater force for change than a person who has healed themselves. They are powerful.

This is what I call Radical Health.

Cellular Healing – Physical Actions

The basic premise with cellular restoration and healing is to think natural. Nature is restorative. Eat hydrating foods and get hydrated through good water. The saying goes, 'Eat, drink and bathe' in what nourishes the cells.

Balance the pH in your body by alkalising. This means a predominantly organic whole food diet and detoxification of the whole system (more on this in a later chapter).

Get your lymph system moving by exercise, lymph tissue drainage (massage), fruits (particularly berries, grapes, melon).

Oxygenate the body, make sure your vitamin and mineral levels are good. If not take supplements.

Drink the best water you can find. Not only filtered but activated in some way.

Nourish with Essential Fatty Acids, the healthy oils.

Lighten the toxic load, meaning really look at what you are absorbing and take radical action to reduce the load wherever you can.

Sleep and rest, relaxation and pleasure are essential to cellular health.

Cellular Healing – Conscious Actions

Think nourishment through healing thoughts and calming emotions.

Bring subconscious beliefs that may be stressing the cells to the surface for healing.

Practice meditations and visualisations for cellular healing.

Understand where you feel disconnected from parts of yourself, other people or the world, and let this disconnection be healed.

Remove disharmony. Remove stress.

Take radical healing action based on profound intuitive intelligence.

Take dominion over your world as a benevolent king or queen. Take back your power and use it as a force for good in both your inner kingdom and in the world.

See yourself as healed and whole. Drop all notion of fragmentation as no longer relevant.

You are designed to be in harmony from the smallest part to the biggest, from the densest to the lightest and from the grossest to the most subtle. To step into your birthright, whether you are ill or not, requires conscious effort. Most people are not prepared to make that effort. Those who do are split into two camps: those that are not ill, and those that are. Illness is a great motivator for those who seize the opportunity. If you are in that camp then I encourage you to take charge of your healing, from the cellular level to the mental, emotional and spiritual. It all fits together eventually and becomes one. To feel in a state of harmony is the most blessed feeling in the world. To be connected to the earth beneath and the heavens above is the most natural feeling in the world. It is a sad thing that most people never feel it.

If you are in the 'not ill' camp, I implore you to seek greater harmony and follow some of these tips anyway. I have seen so many people believe they are immune to illness and convince themselves they are almost immortal. (I was one of these once.) It is simply not true. Your insurance policy is to keep your cells clean and in a healthy environment, so feed your inner body healthy, vibrant and loving foods, thoughts and emotions, and prevent any dis-ease entering your system. Do it the easy way, don't wait until there is some breakdown.

I go into more detail in the next chapter **'Cellular Rehydration and Fasting.'**

Recommended reading:
Cellular Awakening by **Barbara Wren**
Biology of Belief by **Bruce Lipton**

CELLULAR REHYDRATION THROUGH FASTING

Most people are dehydrated on the cellular level. Unless you have paid attention through your life to this fundamental issue and taken consistent action, your diet, lifestyle and emotions will have left you dehydrated.

The chances are that some, if not all, of your digestive tract is clogged up with old, undigested food matter. This can be in the large colon, where most cleansing effort is focused, or it can be in the more complex, thinner and longer small intestine. The small intestine is harder to clean than the large. A colonic hydrotherapy, for example, can only reach to the top of the large intestine, the ileocecal valve, but can get no further. When digestion in the stomach is impaired, as it is with many people, undigested and improperly broken down foodstuff, that which is harder to break down like meat, passes into the small intestine for further breakdown and extraction of nutrients. If the small intestine is in any way compromised and blocked, the process of maximum absorption is impeded.

It is the beginning of a potential cascade of issues that grow gradually over the years. It is also where cellular dehydration begins and ends.

If absorption is restricted AND the diet is improperly biased towards dry, processed, fried, heavily salted foods there is simply no way that the cells in your body are going to get enough hydration.

Some have said that cellular dehydration is the root cause of the majority of chronic diseases.

And it really comes down to how clean the entire digestive tract is, from mouth to anus. If the pipes aren't clean the system is clogged, any plumber will tell you that.

If your system is dehydrated, at some point it's going to start stealing water to keep the vital organs in stasis. That means taking water from what the body intelligence considers non-essential places, eyes, joints and extremities. This level of dehydration is serious and affects the whole organism.

If the cells are dehydrated, they are not able to function. They cannot perform their daily operations from night to day of exchanging sodium and calcium (daytime) to potassium and magnesium (night-time). Small amounts of sodium deposits stay in the cells, increasing dehydration even further. Under these conditions cells cannot eliminate effectively. And the 'poop' from each cell is not carried away conclusively by the lymph system, and hey presto we are creating the ideal conditions for cancer, arthritis, major bowel disorders, brain malfunctions, and other systemic dis-eases.

So just drink more water yeah?

I'm afraid it's not that easy. Simply drinking more water doesn't appear to work very well. You are probably still eating regularly like everyone else. That is your body's priority, digestion, absorption, elimination. It takes up the whole day with its complex activity. It's going to find it hard to do something else also. It will also just allow most water to pass right through the system without going anywhere. Of course it will help a bit, and if it's excellent water that is a big plus. But it is very hard to get enough hydration down to the cellular level through the clogged up pipes. This is why juice fasting and raw food living on fresh watery produce are so popular, they really help.

And most definitely eating an abundance of juicy ripe fruits like papaya and melon helps considerably, in fact for many people this is a great place to start. And of course salads.

But fasting gets to the root of the issue, when supported and effectively executed.

Put simply, extended fasts mean the body no longer has to turn its attention to digesting daily intake. And that simple fact means it can turn its focus to the stuff that lives in the body that shouldn't be there. In essence it is that simple. Drinking water on a fast allows the body to begin the process of absorbing it into the dried up matter lodged deep in the small and large intestine. It takes time, depending on how long it has been there and how dried up it is.

The Power of Illness

There are scores of other benefits to be gained from fasting, but for our purposes we will focus on this central issue.

Having completed a 21-day water fast, I can testify to all the above. Of course the digestive fire goes out during a fast, and elimination all but stops, but it is after the fast that things can happen. If you have maintained a decent level of hydration, then at the end, when you break the fast and during the re-feeding program, which is a vital part of the fast, all sorts of stuff can come out. Reports from those who run fasting centres are that is extremely common to go through this deep toxic elimination. And the stuff seems to come from both the small and large intestine. Some of the utterly dried up matter can go back decades. It might be black and dry. It took one guy, I was told, three hours of toilet sitting to get some of the stuff out. And it's not just once, it can happen every day as more and more is loosened. Quite frankly, it is genius.

The water from the bulk of the fast does some of the job of getting fluid where it needs to go, but then the water from juicy fruits that are used to break the fast, specifically papaya, water melon, cantaloupe melon and coconut water, all in increasing amounts, are the water the body loves best, and it uses them well. By the third day, the peristaltic movement should kick in and then the body eliminates.

The program I took part in was a 21-day fast on water and then a week of re-feeding on small amounts of the fruits mentioned above, plus a small salad after a few days. Then we were encouraged to follow at minimum a six-week protocol of the same basic extremely hydrating fruits and salad. (I give details of the fasting retreat centre in the Useful Resources section of this book.)

This becomes the way we rehydrate the cellular body. And it makes a difference to health in a profound way. Skin clears up and tightens, fuzzy head clears up, replaced by clarity of consciousness. Energy sky rockets to a new level. Building muscle becomes easier, as does all exercise. Flexibility improves enormously. Creativity sparkles. Digestion and elimination improve enormously. The long term of effects of a water fast conducted and broken appropriately, for the right person, can impact and improve the quality of life incredibly. All aspects of health will be affected for the better. If you take care of your diet after the fast you can expect to feel the benefits for years.

Of course if you simply do the fast and then return to toxic behaviours the effect will be short lived.

Fasting is an opportunity. I talk about opportunities we are graced with much of the time as you may have noticed. Simply because I truly believe we are being offered these rare gifts all the time, but fail to notice them under the weight of our neurosis and preoccupation with our concerns.

And fasting is a challenge, of that there is no doubt. But courage and trust are our two best allies when it comes to this kind of experience. We have two choices:

1. We listen to the nay-sayers who cast doubt on anything that is outside what the mainstream knows and

approves of. This tactic throws us off from any possibility of following our own intuition and intelligence and turns us into mindless followers of something we may not even believe in. We will never know what we actually believe in because it has already been decided for us.

2. We follow the path less trodden into the mystery of life, taking our fears with us, but knowing that we trust ourselves and our intelligence. We step out, alone if necessary, as a warrior might, and face whatever comes. We are in danger of living in homogenous societies where individuality is all but ruled out.

Water fasting is one of those practices that has its roots in the oldest of cultures dating back thousands of years. Jesus fasted for forty days and nights, seeking cleansing and power. Mohammed, when asked, said, *"Everything hath a gateway and the gateway of heaven is fasting."* Fasting was an integral part of training to enter Wisdom School in Ancient Greece. Its everywhere, but like many ancient techniques and practices, it has been dismissed by our science-based thinking.

My personal experience of water fasting led me to realise the utter simplicity of the process is what confounds professionals and public alike. We have grown so used to adding more things when there is a problem, we do not trust the body intelligence to take over the job of healing. So we take pills, pharmaceuticals, supplements by the score, add this food and take away that food, increase this exercise and take this smoothie, but the last thing we try is good old NOTHING!

When an animal in the wild is sick, it crawls away somewhere and stops everything and waits. It either heals or dies, and probably most of the time it heals. The human body is a vast interconnected system of bewildering intelligence. If only we can get out of the way long enough, stop endlessly putting stuff in to keep it busy and give it the chance to deeply rest and cleanse, it will deliver. That is not just my theory, but is testimonial from those who have seen thousands of fasters in many years. I have researched this and found it to be true. The body will heal when it is allowed to and supported, in a sensible and monitored environment.

I don't advise doing a fast longer than ten days on your own. You need support and daily monitoring to check your vital signs, particularly if you are ill. Fasting is not a throw-away idea. It is a serious undertaking that needs deep consideration and consultation. But if it draws you in, the benefits can be enormous.

Fasting can possibly help these conditions:

- Diabetes
- Cardiovascular disease
- Inflammatory bowel disease
- Osteo and Rheumatoid arthritis
- Candida and leaky gut
- Epilepsy

- Psychosomatic disease
- Eczema
- Fibromyalgia
- Ulcers
- Circulatory disease
- Asthma
- Depression and Anxiety
- Addiction
- Parasites
- Fibroids
- MS
- Brain fog

CLEAN THE TEMPLE

Cleanliness is next to Godliness

As I have said before, your body is the temple in which you welcome and pray to God consciousness. It is a sacred interface with the world, where consciousness and experience mingle. Having free will means we get to choose how we live in our temple, and how we look after it. Do we treat it with respect and love it and shower it with prayers? Is it our sacred garden? Or do we treat it like a profane dumping ground and live carelessly?

There is no doubting that a heavily toxic overburdened body is going to find it harder to welcome the divine than a light detoxified one. Being toxic and laden with chemicals dominates thought and emotion, it is all consuming, and weighs heavily.

The body can be dense or light depending on what it has to carry. It carries ALL our unprocessed and suppressed emotions and thoughts. It carries and stores everything it cannot let go of, and that means we become the storage container for years of old 'stuff.' Most of it has been forgotten yet it still lives unconsciously inside us as physical toxicity, but also as habitual trigger points in certain situations. It is what Eckhart Tolle calls the pain body. Tolle approaches this from the spiritual level, but what happens when someone has manifested dis-ease? Is it enough to approach it spiritually, or do we need to also include some healing of the body?

Add to this the enormous toxic load the modern human is under and how that load interferes with the human experience, and you will see that cleaning the body temple is not just a great idea but actually a vital thing to do for overall wellbeing and treatment of any dis-ease. Don't underestimate the power of cleansing to create radical shifts on all levels of being. Detox will change your experience of the world if done right. It will lighten the load and ease the burden you carry through life.

In this chapter I am going to talk about two areas: the gut (by gut I mean the whole digestive system but focusing on the colon), and the liver. There are many other areas that we can cleanse, nourish and heal (kidneys, adrenals, lungs, heart and brain for example) but my direct experience is with these two areas and I know how powerful they are, so we are going to focus our attention here.

I absolutely know that my current good health has its roots in the Panchakarma processes I did 2004-2008. My body was wracked by toxins from years of drug abuse. The acidic residue of these dangerous chemical compounds (like amphetamine sulphate) had buried itself deep in the cells of my body, in tissues, organs and joints. My poor liver had taken a pounding from the drugs and alcohol and I was slowly sliding into chronic illness. Thank God for Ayurveda and the opportunity to remove some of the 'hot stuff' that was causing such problems. But it meant I had to go to India to do it.

Strangely, although we live in the sickest, most toxic societies in the history of mankind, we are still totally inept at removing toxins and dealing with chronic illness. We should be masters in this, yet we are utterly useless. In fact, if you go to your medical doctor today and talk about detoxification of your body or their thoughts on a liver cleanse you will get the same blank look as when you talk to them about diet. Nothing comes back at you. They are simply not trained in detox or diet so they do not recognise it. They will say nothing or they will try and talk you out of it by saying it is unnecessary or dangerous. They are trained in diagnosis, symptomatology, medication and surgical treatment, anything beyond this remit is incomprehensible.

But many old cultures and religions have used cleansing and detox as part of their accepted rituals. Ayurveda has its Panchakarma treatment, Chinese medicine has developed precise ways of detoxifying internal organs, the old greek wisdom culture spoke of this cleanliness and fasting, Jesus and the Essenes fasted for spiritual and physical purposes. Islam has Ramadan, a month of fasting. Many indigenous cultures used sweat lodges and of course saunas have been popular for centuries. But in our modern western urban world we have nothing. We have no built in way to remove our toxic load. It is a pharmaceutical dream. It means we don't get to renew our physical vehicles and we don't get to connect with our core spiritual essence. We just hurtle along like a car with no brakes.

We can be grateful that a new awareness has arisen in the last decade that has opened the door to modalities and programs that help us detox and heal. They have yet to be embraced by the mainstream as they may well pose a threat to the established pharmaceutical companies, but the march of health wisdom has begun and is becoming unstoppable. People are not only waking up spiritually, they are also waking up physically to what it means to be fully well.

> *The wave of evolution is sweeping through health and spirituality at this time, because they are connected. It's all energy.*

The connection between cleansing the body and spiritual purity is well known. In the '**Gospel of Peace**' Jesus talks of Satan and evil as actually living inside the body. Reading his description is like reading a description of a body infested with parasites, candida, impacted fecal matter and toxins. Jesus, in this revelatory little book, says that cleansing the demons (toxins, worms, etc) from the body is necessary to return it to its natural state. Cleansing realigns the body and brings a cellular flow which calms the mind and reconnects you with the natural order of things.

> *I actually believe it helps release the cellular body from the stranglehold of ego.*

The more I have looked into this area, in research and in deep personal reflection, the more I believe that the cleansing and healing of the cells is fundamental to physical and spiritual health. It is as though this cellular healing allows more light to penetrate the cells, which in turn somehow remaps the DNA itself. This is a profoundly transformative notion!

Cleanliness is next to Godliness

Being overly toxic, acidic or infested with parasites knocks us out of our natural state. Some people may even appear possessed by 'entities.' But these ideas point us to this notion of cleanliness and Godliness. If we take Godliness to mean our natural state of being, the state that connects us to life, each other and spirit, and cleanliness to mean an inner state (not the state of our house) then this profound statement makes perfect sense.

Cleaning our inner temple (our bodies) creates a purification that allows us to physically resonate more naturally. This natural resonance brings a vibration of love, gratitude and compassion and we begin to become humble containers for God's love and wisdom (by 'God' I mean compassionate consciousness).

Natural law is then lived inside us, as us. We become tuned in to life. Our inner state dictates our outer state. This has nothing to do with moral or religious dogma. And nothing to do with God as a bearded guy in the sky. It has to do with the deepest experience of who we are.

A clean vehicle will better embrace divine energy.

Heal Your Gut

A few gut facts:

Your gut holds so much intelligence it's called the second brain.

70% of your immune system is located in your gut.

The gut produces more of the neurotransmitter serotonin than your brain.

Gut bacteria outnumbers cells in your body by 10 to 1.

There are more nerve cells in your enteric nervous system (which includes the gut) than your central nervous system.

We are only just waking up to the importance of the gut in well-being, but we know enough to take action when we need to. And most people need to. Digestive disorders are rising rapidly as is colon cancer and inflammatory bowel dis-ease. Auto immune dis-eases (anything from rheumatoid arthritis to thyroid problems, scleroderma, lupus, etc) are a massive problem, and since the immune system is located mostly in the gut then cleaning up the gut is logical. But apparently this kind of simple logic has not reached as far as mainstream medical health yet.

The US National Library of Medicine lists 80 disorders directly related to Auto-Immune, yet also says that most of these are chronic disorders that have no cure but can be controlled with modern drugs. Once again this is excellent news for the pharmaceutical companies.

So we are on our own. You have to investigate and research for yourself. You have to find natural healers who will help you. There are many colon specialists out there, many naturopaths and Ayurvedic doctors who can offer this kind of cleansing. Or you can do some of this yourself.

If your gut is clogged up and constipated, if you have candida (yeast growth) or leaky gut, you will be mentally out of balance. That is guaranteed. And here is what is most alarming. The modern lifestyle looks almost designed to destroy the entire digestive system, including the gut.

Here is what hits your digestive system and gut: Toxins, pathogens, sugar, wheat, gluten, parasites, caffeine, free radicals, medications, chemicals, antibiotics, steroids, antacids, electromagnetic frequency emissions from mobile phones, wireless towers and cordless phones, and dirty electricity, fungus, processed foods, colourings, undigested non-organic meat, and of course, buried emotions and stress.

This modern living is driving us crazy, and the only way to cope with it is to de-stress and detox, put nutrients in and flood the body with goodness.

If it's not flowing through from mouth to anus then it's getting stuck somewhere. It needs to be healthy from the top to the bottom. You have a big tube running through your body. This tube is the opening to the external world and it needs to run efficiently. At the mouth stage it chews and swallows food. Proper mastication is vital to the subsequent process, but is all too often overlooked by the 'gulp and go' lifestyle. The stomach, already alerted (hopefully) to the type of food it expects, greets food with the acids necessary to break it down into usable form. Off it shuffles to the small intestine for the big job of absorption of nutrients. And then it goes to the large intestine for final removal of moisture and readying for return to the outside world as waste product. It's a highly complex process that can mess up pretty easily and it needs your support. It's your link to life. Right now it's the best one you have. No food means no life. No absorption means you waste away. No elimination means the backing up of fecal matter.

Weak digestive process equals weak absorption equals weak elimination. That means life force is reduced, susceptibility to outside threats increases, from virus to fungus, and we don't have enough power to fight them off. It is a spiral downhill unless we maintain digestive and gut health.

Maintaining awareness of the process actually connects us with it. It is not a food processing machine it's a highly evolved sophisticated process that needs care, attention and love. Treated well and loved it will be strong and robust. Abused, neglected and taken for granted it will fall into disrepair.

Here is my list of recommendations:

- Chew your food well, let your stomach know it is on its way. The beginning of the process is as important as the end. Take smaller bites, and put the fork down between mouthfuls. Develop calmness as your default eating style.

- Turn off the radio, the tv, and cease as much chat as possible. It all distracts from the digestion. Relax into silence when you eat.

- Make sure your digestive fire is strong but not burning too hot. Millions of people suffer from weak or over active digestive fire and take antacids for it. This is an unnecessary act and a disaster for health and wellbeing. Help your digestive fire with apple cider vinegar or some fresh ginger and lemon juice. It's ok to use some good quality digestive enzymes. I have used papaya enzymes and they are very effective.

- Cut out the indigestible foods. Wheat, gluten, processed foods, dairy (unless its raw), soy, corn, synthetic sugars, grains, trans fats, preservatives, and soft fizzy drinks.

- Get checked for candida. If you have candida then follow the candida clearing diet. I recommend **Donna Gates** 'Body Ecology Diet.' There are thousands of online resources for getting tested. This in itself is very important. Both candida and leaky gut are primary markers for systemic problems that, unless dealt with at source, multiply and deepen. They don't just go away, they need to be sent packing. Incidentally I have to confess a few years ago when I heard about candida I thought it was just a woman's problem, and even then I didn't actually believe in it. I do now. It is real and it compromises health seriously and chronically.

- Check for leaky gut. If you do then follow candida diet. There are thousands of on line resources for getting tested. I'm certain I suffered from chronic leaky gut, but never got tested. If the barrier of the gut has been breached, it means proteins and other unwanted guests are penetrating areas of the body they just shouldn't be, like the blood stream. It could be this activity that triggers what we call the auto-immune response. So going back and clearing up the gut, healing the lining with diet and herbs makes complete sense.

- Check for parasites. Most people imagine that parasites, worms and fungus only happen in the poor Asian countries, but that myth is ridiculous. Millions of americans and english citizens are infested with unwanted guests. When there are gut issues this may well be the case, but not just with gut issues. If you think this may be you then a parasite cleanse is very worthwhile and beneficial. It must be thorough and involve cloves, wormwood and black walnut hull. The protocol is online and well-researched. The expert to follow is **Dr Hulda Clark** (www.drclark.net)

- Colon Cleanse! There is no doubt in my mind about the benefits of colon cleansing. A course of professional colon cleanses will clear out old gunk and help

the colon wall to breathe. This one act alon[e]
all the difference. If you are completely [unsure]
of colon cleanse then find something calle[d]
Colosan is a magnesium-based colon cleansing product that you take orally, and it is very effective. Of course you can do enemas at home, all you need to buy is an enema bag, easily available at a chemist, and follow the procedure easily found online. But home enemas only get so far into the lower intestine. A series of colonics with a professional would be an excellent gift to give yourself. This is very probably the first place I would start. And I would not wait until I was ill. Everyone should do it.

Extra considerations: These are things I have used or do use. The list is by no means extensive but it gives some idea of the number of ways you can assist colon and gut health.

Digestive Enzymes to assist digestion, **Fermented foods** (making these yourself is easy and very satisfying), **Raw milk**, **Apple Cider Vinegar**, **Wheatgrass**, **Chlorella**, **Chlorophyll**, **L-Glutamine**, **Raw Coconut Oil**, **Green tea**.

Fresh Juices. We are living in the days of the great juice revolution. Buy a juicer and get juicing. This single act could catapult your health to another dimension!

Bitters, **Ginger** to stimulate digestion.

Fennel, **Cardamom**, **Cumin**, **Coriander**, and **Caraway** to aid digestion.

Slippery Elm, **Chia Seeds**, **Flax Seeds** for moisture, fibre and mucilage in the bowel.

Good quality **Probiotics** are becoming a necessity for living in todays anti biotic world.

Curcumin, **Raw Turmeric Root** for inflammation and digestion. Turmeric is considered to be an almost divine healing spice it has so many extraordinary healing qualities.

The Squatty Potty! The single most beneficial asset to your toilet. We are not designed to sit, we are designed to squat. Sitting pinches the bowel, squatting opens it. This simple addition helps elimination, constipation and all gut-related issues. Seriously, buy one, you will not regret it.

Intermittent Fasting. Recent experiments show that daily fasting helps the body in quite amazing ways. To be effective, in the case of daily intermittent fasting, the length of your fast must be at least 16 hours. This means eating only between the hours of 11am until 7pm, as an example. Essentially, this equates to simply skipping breakfast, and making lunch your first meal of the day instead.

We actually skip the evening meal, finishing eating at 2.30pm and then having breakfast at about 8am. It is very much an individual lifestyle decision.

It is valuable for fat burning, and building Human Growth Hormone (HGH), gives the digestive system a rest, boosts metabolism, reduces inflammation and lessens free radical damage, normalises insulin and leptin sensitivity, which is key for optimal health.

Added to high-intensity interval training, this is the current model many people are using to create excellent health, boost muscle growth and take well-being to a new level.

Heal your Liver

> *"The physician who knows how to harmonise the liver knows how to treat a hundred diseases."* - **Zhou Xuehai**, *Reflections Upon Reading the Medical Classics (Du Yi Suibi), ca. 1895*

I have been doing a lot of research into the role of the liver in dis-ease and health recently and I can honestly say that healing this overloaded organ is vital to wellbeing. Whether you choose to do a liver flush itself or take the more systematic and slow journey in many ways doesn't matter. What matters is attending to it, and giving it some love and nourishment will give you energy, radiance and peace.

A few facts:

Liver dis-ease is UK's 5th biggest killer.

28% of people tested showed early signs of liver damage.

Twice as many people now die from liver dis-ease than in 1991.

In the last three years alone there has been an increase in liver dis-ease deaths by 12%!

It is increasing at a staggering rate, and now kills more people than diabetes and road deaths combined.

Liver dis-ease frequently causes multiple organ dysfunction, so the true statistics could be much higher.

And quite honestly when you understand what we are taking into our bodies you will not be surprised.

It is not just alcohol that hurts the liver. It is, as we shall see, an organ under assault from the modern world. It is an organ, the second largest organ of your body, that works very hard for you. It has so many functions it is incredible. The liver filters over a litre of blood every minute. It is responsible for detoxifying, nourishing, replenishing and storing blood. Wait a minute! Did I read that right? It's responsible for the blood? If blood is acidic or contaminated or below optimal strength then illness and even death will surely follow. And the liver will never allow the blood to become acidic so it works and works and works to maintain balance. But it cannot go on forever, unless you help it.

It is important for hormone regulation. Interestingly, it is also our weight controlling organ. It removes dead cells, cancer cells and toxins. It converts fat soluble chemicals and toxins into water soluble substances and prepares them for elimination through skin, urine, saliva or the GI tract. The liver generates energy and heat. It is the protector of the Immune system. In Chinese medicine the liver is the 'mother' of the heart.

An over-worked, stagnant or heavily toxic liver is implicated in many dis-eases: Obesity, diabetes, cirrhosis, cancer, auto-immune dis-ease, inflammation, infections, allergies, chronic fatigue, fibromyalgia, skin dis-ease, migraines and digestive issues.

The liver has to process, isolate and eliminate all the chemicals and toxins we eat, breathe, and absorb through our skin that are a threat to health. Many of these are carcinogenic, and that means that if your liver is not functioning at full capacity because of past burdens, it is just not going to be up to the job. I know many people, particularly the medical profession but not only them, think that the liver takes care of itself and should not be interfered with, but with the sheer volume of chemicals and toxins in today's world that is, to say the least, naive.

The modern urban human is a walking experiment in toxic overload. We are all in uncharted territory, guinea pigs in the laboratory called the modern world. And unless we are taking active care of our wellbeing, supporting our besieged bodies and making conscious healthy choices, we could easily fall foul of this experiment.

Chemical and Toxic Load

Since the Second World War more than 80,000 new chemicals have been invented. 4 billion pounds of toxic chemicals are released into the global environment each year, 72 million of which are known carcinogens. Many of these chemicals have not been tested for their impact on human health. Since the dawn of the 20th Century, modern agriculture, war and increased industrialisation have arrived with blessings and curses. The curse of the modern way of life is that it is killing us, slowly but surely, and will continue to do so until we acknowledge this and take creative action. And that will mean minimising the amount of chemical pollution in every area of life.

Experiment

Take a good look around wherever you are right now. If you are sitting in the middle of nature surrounded by trees and green, then I congratulate you, you are unique. But I will guarantee that most people reading this will be in a chemical laden environment. Look at what you are surrounded by: carpets, wall paint, bed linen, mattress, all toxic to your liver. In the bathroom, body and face products, hair and bath products unless they are 100% natural organic, tend to be laced with chemicals, some of which are carcinogenic. In the kitchen it's the same, non stick pans, toxic washing up liquid and clothes wash, microwave, canned goods, plastic containers. You see, before we even discuss what chemicals you may be eating and drinking that your liver has to deal with, you are already under attack, in your own home!

I'm not trying to scare you, I'm trying to open your eyes. When your eyes are open you can make conscious choices. Avoiding reality doesn't make it go away. It just means you suffer more.

Emotions and Liver Health

The liver is the organ of anger, heat and irritation. It is fiery. Prolonged anger can lead to an imbalance of the liver. At the same time, a liver imbalance can produce symptoms of anger and irritation, setting up a vicious self-perpetuating cycle. Those red faced, hot, fiery people may have an imbalance of the liver. And if liver fire rises too much, the spleen can suffer, producing lack of appetite, indigestion and even diarrhoea.

I used to have the 'hottest' body of anyone I ever met (of course I mean in terms of temperature)! My Chinese doctors were astonished at how much heat I was generating. In the last couple of years before I started doing something about it, I was actually burning up. I have already told you I had rosacea on my face, boils and eruptions. But I also had fainting episodes, headaches, fuzzy thinking, mood swings, anger, irritation and high levels of stress. I can now see just how damaged my liver was. One of the first healers I saw, now a famous natural healer in London who worked for many months on me, said my liver was a mess and would take a long time to heal. And it is true, it has taken time.

But as I have said before, if I can do it, anyone can!

If you experience any of these signs, then you may have a sluggish or toxic liver:

Mood swings, anger and irritation, stress, fatigue, circulation issues, digestive disturbance, allergies, pre menstrual tension, constipation, arthritis, tendon problems, weak or brittle nails, skin problems, bitter taste in mouth, dry or burning eyes.

What can you do?

First, you can change your diet, remove some of the more damaging foods and introduce foods that heal and support your liver health. Remove processed foods, processed sugars, anything with preservatives, anything with GMO, avoid alcohol, remove trans fats, and monitor prescription drugs (thats right, all prescription drugs are toxic to the liver, they are synthetic and intensely chemical and as such are foreign to the body, so the liver is always impacted by medication).

Liver nourishing and detoxifying foods, herbs and spices:

Whole plant foods, mostly raw, fruits and veg, berries, lemons, melons and grapes, specifically cruciferous veg (brussel sprouts, broccoli, cauliflower), squash, sweet potato, green leafy veg, beetroot, carrots, onions, garlic. Walnuts, avocado, asparagus, raw tomatoes, grapefruit, lean protein... and only small amounts.

Herbs and spices: Turmeric and its derivative curcumin, mustard seed, caraway seed, spearmint, oregano, sweet basil, cilantro, milk thistle, dandelion, ginger, burdock.

Specifics: Seaweed, kelp, grape seed extract, zinc, magnesium, selenium, flax oil, hemp oil, chia seeds, coconut oil, oily fish, bitters.

Vitamins and minerals: Zinc, magnesium, selenium, vitamin D, E and A, glutathione, essential fatty acids, taurine, alpha lipoic acid.

Consider a Liver and Gallbladder Cleanse: Not everyone is in favour of taking this kind of action, believing that it is unnecessary as the liver is already trying to detox. If you are drawn to this intuitively and want to pursue it, I recommend the **Andrea Moritz** 'Liver and Gallbladder Flush.' It is well researched and the process is described very clearly. Many thousands of people have done it and reported excellent results, and much better health as a result. I have tried it twice and prefer something a little more gentle as it seems to impact my sensitive colon a bit too much. My wife loves it! There are options for everyone. You can take the slow road or the fast road, some of which will depend on the urgency of your situation.

Give your liver a rest! It detoxifies at night so don't overload with lots of heavy, fatty food, before you go to bed! Eat early, eat light, and get as much digestion finished as possible so your body is actually resting. This will help your liver to do its job more thoroughly. If you are waking up in the night at 2am your liver is being overworked. If you are also hot upon waking at that time your liver needs your help.

Emotionally: This really is a 'chicken and egg' situation. If you can really deal with the anger, irritation and stress in your life, it will calm your liver down and allow it to heal. Conversely if you take some of the steps above and actively support liver health, your anger, irritation and stress will slowly decline, and you will find yourself less hot and bothered. If you take both actions, something transformational will happen!

Other actions to take: Some of these ideas are long term actions in your house. Don't be put off by the magnitude of the task, just be systematic, one thing at a time. The main thing is: think natural and organic. All synthetic products carry chemicals, and those chemicals leach into skin and lungs, and your home is probably full of synthetic products. So go natural. In your bathroom throw out the toxic toothpaste and shampoo. Avoid any body products you can't eat, particularly those with parabens, sodium lauryl sulphate or oxybenzone. Choose only organic natural toxin-free body and face products. Make your own cleaning products. Get an organic mattress when you can (we haven't got one yet but one day we will). Get natural paint, natural carpets, natural clothes, natural bed linen. Avoid wifi anywhere near the bedroom.

The results of cleaning up and supporting your liver: You could benefit in many ways, here are some possibilities. Skin conditions decrease or disappear, blood sugar stabilises, mind becomes clear, heat disappears from body, better digestion, mood stabilises, anger decreases, better fat metabolism (which means losing weight), high blood pressure reduction, decreased cancer risk, more energy, reduction in inflammation, improved immune system function, auto immune symptoms begin to disappear.

Conclusion

So there you have it, two areas you can get to work on right now. Loving your liver and caring for your colon will bring such dividends you cannot imagine right now. What I have offered is a brief glimpse into the possibilities taking care of your inner body will offer you. There is extensive information available on the web, and book ideas I have listed at the end. If in any doubt find a professional natural practitioner who can help in these areas. And working on the physical body at the same time as diving into emotions is very powerful, so be prepared for ups and downs. Whenever we start to dislodge what has been stuck for many years, it releases the emotion for healing. It is all energy to be embraced and allowed.

SOME WORDS ABOUT RAW FOOD

I am not here to tell you what is right or wrong when it comes to eating raw food. There are so many arguments out there, so many disagreements, that I just cannot add yet another pro or anti raw voice to it. The truth is that over the last few years I have, at times, been fully raw, semi-raw and even not raw at all. And I have come to the conclusion that these things are nebulous. Every single person on this planet has a unique blueprint and footprint. We have evolved to adapt to many things, and we have been influenced by many factors.

For a start we have different body types. We have different sizes, shapes, metabolism and characters. We have a very different ancestry from each other. Consider the difference between an Eskimo and a Hawaiian. Or the difference between a Chinese man and a Norwegian man. They are (mostly) structurally different, they have different tendencies and different physiologies. How can we apply a 'one size fits all' diet when it's obvious how different we are? And when it comes to eating we are not all the same. For thousands of years Indian culture has been predominantly vegetarian. It's a hot country. Eskimo culture is predominantly fish and blubber. It's a cold climate. You are the inheritor of a genetic adaptation to the environment. And you have inherited certain weaknesses and strengths handed down through your family genealogy and very much from your father and mother. On top of this you were very impacted by the state of health of your mother during pregnancy and the early months of your birth. This makes you a unique individual with unique needs. You do not fit into a box, and that means you have to follow your own inner guidance system in all things, including what works food-wise.

Just because someone eats a healthy diet, it may not actually heal them or create well-being, because there are so many subtle factors involved in creating health or recovering from illness that, despite their best efforts to 'do the right thing,' it just may not happen. All we are really doing is increasing the odds, but there is never a guarantee in life. I have known people who have eaten raw food and their health has gone down hill after the initial burst of energy and cleansing. I know people who thrive on the diet. I know people who desperately want to be raw but it just doesn't work for them, for whatever reason. I know people who eat cooked food (particularly the Ayurvedic diet) who are as well as anyone I have seen. So I have dropped the idea that raw is best in favour of a much more flexible approach to food.

Having said that, there are certain principles that are fundamental, whether you are choosing raw food, cooked food, meat food or a combination. So before I talk about my own experience with raw, let me lay some of these basic principles out. You probably already do this but if you don't consider these options:

- **ALWAYS** choose organic natural foods wherever possible.

- **ALWAYS** include fresh fruits and veg in your diet.

- **REMOVE** as much of the processed, canned and dead food from your kitchen as you dare. You are aiming to have none!

- **DO NOT EAT**: Processed sugar, artificial sweeteners, processed salt, any food with an additive, any food with a preservative, canned tomatoes, processed meat, margarine or vegetable oils.

- **THINK** ,'Is this food as natural as it can be?' If it is, eat it.

- **DO NOT EAT GMO FOOD.**

My experience with Ayurveda and Raw Food

If you don't know about Ayurveda and you want to understand some fundamentals about body and personality types, I recommend investing a little time reading about it. There is just too much to go into here. For a quick general overview read this:

http://medical-dictionary.thefreedictionary.com/Ayurvedic+medicine

In Ayurveda I am a vata type, and a classic one. I am prone to coldness, anxiety, being too 'mindy,' but also creative and changeable. I am excitable and artistic and can talk way too fast. My energy is all there one minute and gone the next. I get easily over stimulated and pay the price. I use up my energy fast and don't have much on back up so have a tendency to depletion. I can get ungrounded easily. I am prone to addictions and have difficulty sleeping. I can multi-task when I'm balanced but become scattered when I'm out of whack. When I am out of balance my moods can change like the weather, and the weather affects me greatly. Worst seasons for me are the dry and cold autumn and winter. Vata types can experience lower back pain (yes), joint pain (yes), and colon problems (yes).

My task is to get vata balanced and calm through regularity and routine, good sleeping and nourishing foods. In Ayurveda raw food is contra indicated as it is much too cold and indigestible. They favour warming, oily and soupy foods.

Remember this as I now talk about my journey into raw.

The first part of my healing journey, when I met Amoda and during the 3 Panchakarmas, was all supported by an Ayurvedic diet. The diet is, in its essence, a healing one, with very specific recipes for specific actions in the body, and using the many spices and herbs of India. I responded very well to this food as long as I didn't overdo the rice. But we didn't have much salad, and no fruit at all! Neither of us knew anything about the raw food 'movement' as it was still very new and almost unheard of in the UK. We discovered raw food and superfoods in 2008 when Amoda was on a trip to the US. We had already experimented with the pH Miracle protocol and the whole principle of alkalising so we were ready for what was to come.

Raw foods, which means whole plant foods, vegetables and fruits eaten in their uncooked state, are extremely cleansing and powerful. They are highly nutritious and flood the body with vitality and water.

But they are challenging on digestion and the digestive system for some people. Most people come to raw food with damaged digestive fire and compromised digestion. Raw food is cooling, and needs stronger digestive juices to break down in the stomach and small intestine. There is a lot more cellulose fibre to process and the pre-cooking action has just been eliminated.

Imagine, most people have been eating predominantly cooked food all their lives. They may have included salads here and there, but the vast majority of their diet has been cooked. Their digestion has grown used to this so has actually adapted to it and come to expect it. One day everything changes, and now the food arrives in the stomach uncooked, tough, in it's pristine raw state. Much as we like to think that the body is super intelligent and adaptable, it is also slow and gets stuck in a rut. It just doesn't have the fire power, the strong juices and acids, to suddenly meet this revolution of raw food arriving in the stomach. It will cope. It may make some noise, it may impact digestion and elimination. It may cause gas and bloating, but it will do the job, kind of. Remember, if digestion is wrong, the whole process suffers. If digestion is wrong, absorption is compromised. If absorption is compromised, elimination will be inconclusive.

But you may not notice for a while.

The positive effects will outweigh the negative. Your body will extract what it can and flood your cells with oxygen, water, vitamins, minerals, whole food nutrition and light. It will lift your energy and detox your body. The introduction of this fibrous, water rich, mineral dense, cooling green food will begin its cleansing process, and for some, particularly the vata types, this may well begin to aggravate the dosha. The last thing the vata type needs is cooling down, they are already cold!

And if you have an already compromised immune system (inflammatory bowel dis-ease is considered an immune system problem), or if you suffer from adrenal fatigue or problematic kidneys, the cooling, cleansing effect can be dramatic.

Now, at this point I would say that if you are living in a warm climate like California or Hawaii then this cooling problem is not such an issue, but if you are living in the United Kingdom or most other cold, damp and cloudy climates, it's going to be tough going. So many raw food 'gurus' say you can be raw anywhere in the world, and in theory thats true, but in reality its just not that simple.

We lived predominantly raw for the next few years. We were in Somerset UK, a cold and damp environment, in a chilly house and I was recovering from chronic illness and trying to build strength and health. But although I was getting clearer and clearer and more and more enthusiastic about the new raw diet, I was actually getting colder and colder. My immune system just wasn't getting the warming food support it needed.

The excitement of the raw food revolution over ruled my body intelligence. Body was screaming, 'Give me something warm!' but mind was saying, 'This raw diet is so high vibration and has such a cleansing effect it's got to be good!' so I just ignored the growing problem, thinking it would all be alright.

I thought raw food was the answer to everything. I actually became quite radical and felt as though I was in an elite club of special people who had discovered the big secret to eternal life. I held on to this belief, even to the detriment of my health. I honestly couldn't face the fact that my body needed some warm, soupy foods. I thought it needed more cleansing, and that is one of the traps it is easy to fall into. It's not just about cleansing and detoxifying, its also about building the body up and nourishing it with vital nutrients, minerals and sustenance.

To conclude the story, I somehow, with my compromised immune system and living in a mouldy, cold and damp house, contracted fungus and mould in my fingers.

Over two years my immune system collapsed, my finger nails got infected, I had to have two of them lanced for the infection, five of my finger nails fell out, I absolutely froze to the point of crying, I developed Raynaud's syndrome and I developed under active thyroid (Hashimotos). I thought I was dying. In desperation I went to see a Chinese doctor and he told me, among other things, I needed warm foods. This time I listened and acted.

Just for the record I am not saying all this was caused by raw food. In some ways it doesn't interest me what caused what. It was, in my view, all part of the journey and inevitable. My immune system was weak anyway, and the house we lived in was very cold, damp and mouldy, so very possibly I would have got the fungus anyway. It doesn't matter. I am not trying to put raw food down, I am just trying to discuss all sides of the matter. The fact is I love raw foods.

When I started on the warm foods I got stronger and warmer. When I then felt strong enough to do weight training to build muscle and raise my metabolism then things changed dramatically and I began to feel grounded and strong. I imagined that by going back on cooked foods all my health would be lost. Cooked food definitely has a more addictive quality to it, and it brings out the emotional eater more than raw food. I thought I would give up raw for ever and slip back into bad habits.

But the great news is, it didn't happen! What has happened is that now I have the best of both worlds and that means I have flexibility. I have warm and cooked foods when I feel my body needs them, when its cold and damp and windy in autumn and winter, and then when I'm warm and grounded I veer towards raw, plant based food. I love raw food meals and I love feeling warmly grounded and nourished. It has been an empowering experience and given me freedom to choose. For me now it is about balance. If I have too much cooked food I start to feel stodgy and too heavy. If I have too much raw food at the wrong time I just can't digest it and I get gas, bloating and feel cold, it doesn't nourish me. But if I can successfully navigate between the two then I am on track. It is a day to day experience of listening to my body and feeling into what it wants.

My advice

Don't think in terms of raw versus cooked. Think of what your body needs. Don't be hooked on should and should nots. Tune in, experiment and feel your way. Discover your Ayurvedic dosha type (pitta, vata, kapha). It may help you to understand why you react certain ways.

Eat natural foods, whether you cook them or not.

Always include some fresh green leaves with your food. Upscale the amount of fresh raw that you include depending on season.

Consider the long-game approach to eating raw food. Be systematic and see that in two or three years you will be more raw, and slowly introduce new elements to your diet. This gives your digestive fire and system a chance to adapt. Take digestive enzymes to help this slow transition.

Don't be terrified of raw food, it's one of the best new friends you will have.

Warm up raw food choices with spices. Ginger, Turmeric, Cumin, Coriander, Cayenne, Lemon juice.

Don't be terrified of cooked food, it is an old friend who has looked after you for years.

Don't get hung up and obsessed. Food is not there to get obsessed about. Relax!

Allow digestion to finish before the next meal.

Being 50% - 70% raw is fine.

If you are doubtful, consult a nutritionist in your area.

Monitor the effect on adrenal glands and thyroid, as this is where some of the long term (hidden) damage can take place.

RAW FOOD ADVANTAGES:

This is the potential of the raw food diet. It's not always achievable, but the latent possibility is always here:

Organic raw food is composed of living water and charged particles of electrical potential. The water helps the nutrients enter the cells and both rehydrate them and give them the raw nutrients they need, minerals, vitamins, sugars, proteins, fats and anti oxidants.

It is much more creative and colourful than cooked food.

It gives you heaps of energy.

Raw food diet connects you with life, with the earth.

It is the best diet for detoxification. Each food has a specific action on the body and the innate intelligence of the plants informs your cells, and the cells tell your mind what to do. It becomes an intuitive lifestyle.

At its best raw food living is all about simplicity. It doesn't have to be complex. It can be a glorified salad with a simple but tasty dressing.

You can eat as much as you like! This one takes a bit of getting used to, but it's generally true. As long as it's not just nuts.

The plant cellulose and fruit fibre cleans the intestines and improves elimination.

Raw food helps heal the emotional and mental body bringing clarity and vibrancy.

Raw food is closely associated with the colour of the heart, green. It is the colour of love. It can bring joy and healing. At its best raw food elevates consciousness.

It is the diet of healing.

It is the diet of **peace**. It is, as yet, the least harmful diet to living creatures and the environment.

Raw food is the closest we get to eating light. It is transformed light.

I know this may sound far fetched to some of you, but I feel we will discover in the future that there is a connection between this light and our nourishment which is why the raw revolution has appeared at this time in history. Humanity is going through a massive shake up of consciousness and we are asking fundamental questions about life. As we probe deeper into the nature of reality we are finding more and more mystery.

At the heart of everything is emptiness! This emptiness is not dead but full of potential. And that begs the question, if, at its core, all matter is empty and just full of potential, then what are we being nourished by. Is it really vitamins, minerals, proteins, water and oxygen, or is it light information?

Conclusion

I advocate taking a mature long-view approach to food. It has taken a lifetime to get where you are. If it's urgent, act with urgency, but if it is not, then take your time. Integrate foods, support the body in its actions. Detox but don't suffer. Raw food is not the panacea for everything. Some thrive on it and some suffer. The vata person is going to have a hard time, but that doesn't mean they can't utilise some of the benefits and incorporate them. The pitta person may get on better. But here is also a valuable point. Since I have got stronger and more grounded, and since cleansing my liver more, I have noticed that I am able to tolerate raw foods much better that ever, even in the cold months. The liver and spleen play a big part in this.

The raw food diet is about creating health, vibrancy, space, light, energy, flexibility, love and joy. But if we get too obsessed by having to be a certain way and lose that flexibility then we have defeated the very purpose of it. So stay flexible and, most of all, relax.

THE EVER-EVOLVING DIET

It has been over ten years since my first encounter with the consultant in London and my first experience of the dreaded blood in bowel movements. What a long journey it has been! There has been such an inner evolution on every level of my being, from the physical to the spiritual, that I have always felt myself to be on a mystery path that never ends, but always changes and adapts and grows. My quality of thinking of such matters has been through such a deepening that sometimes I sit back and marvel at the inner dimensions and changes I have been through.

And one of the areas this is reflected in has been, and still is, my diet. I adored Ayurvedic food made by Amoda for many years, and thought I would never change and had come home. We then transitioned to fully raw and Ayurvedic food quickly vanished from our plates. Once again I thought I had reached nirvana and would never change again in my life.

And now recently the evolutionary impulse has changed again and I am finding myself drawn to a high fat diet with reduced carbohydrates.

I have learned not to stay still. Change is the only constant we know, and the body, emotion and mind change their needs. What was relevant once may no longer be relevant. I have missed healthy fats in my diet and now am including them. I eat butter, raw if I can get it, and always from cattle that are grass-fed. I eat eggs, I occasionally eat some fish if it is line caught locally, I eat coconut oil and lots of avocados, some nuts and seeds. I make kefir from locally sourced raw milk and will use full fat cream, also raw.

My leaning right now is towards more paleo diet and high fat, and of course always massive servings of fresh organic salads. I don't eat meat. But I might.

I have read extensively about the 'Real Food' revolution that sits alongside the raw revolution. I was vegetarian and vegan for years and years. Factory farming of any animal is abhorrent.

I also believe we have to make our individual choices and stand by them. I have also researched the whole 'low fat,' high carbohydrate push that happened many years ago and took over the US and British diet world and found it to be fundamentally flawed. The idea that we can thrive without healthy fats looks to me absurd, and the current research is concluding the very same.

We have individual needs. What you need from food might not be what I need. We have different bodies and different metabolic systems. It has even been discovered that there is a variability within the human race in the ration of carbohydrates, proteins and fats needed to create ATP, the energy that powers the body. Some people, it would appear, need more carbohydrates than fats, whereas others need a higher fat to protein to carbohydrate ratio.

And if that balance is wrong, it can lead to a disastrous consequences for health. This is what I have been noticing for myself. I do not thrive well on high carbohydrate diets. I survive but don't get stronger, more muscle, more energy or power. It doesn't feel right. When I eat a high fat and medium protein diet I feel great and I thrive.

David Wolfe had this to say about high carbohydrate diets: *"This is, by far, the most dangerous type of diet. Why? Because statistically it works for the smallest part of the population and for that reason is more likely to cause problems.* (Most people have been convinced that the high carb diet is the only proper diet to eat. Low fat, medium amounts of protein and high carbohydrates) *It is great if you need high carbs in your diet ... but if it's not for you then what can occur is demineralisation."*

The whole area of optimal diet for individual people throws the fox into the chicken coop of the 'one size fits all' diet books and even the raw food dogma. Raw is excellent but it obviously does not work for everyone. I personally do not hold any judgment about whether someone eats meat. We have to find the answers within ourselves.

So what I am really saying is, think smart and keep developing. Keep investigating what works for you and move on. I don't mean from one fad to another, I mean learning to pick out the healthy carbohydrates, and knowing which ones create optimal health, I mean knowing your fats and oils, and knowing (for example) that soaking nuts and seeds vastly increases their digestibility. I mean deciding which protein might be optimal and finding a natural, organic source for it. If you want to drink milk because it really agrees with you, then source raw, grass-fed milk. Constantly refining and redefining your body's needs demands an awareness that keeps you connected to how you feel and how the food you eat makes you feel.

When I consider my journey, I can see this movement ... Twenty years ago I pretty much ate anything, takeaways, kebabs, drank coke and alcohol, didn't care particularly about salad, and hadn't even heard of organic. Things changed and I started eating more salads and fresh food, less processed and cut out the coke. I still ate chocolate bars. And then I kept growing and moved into organic fresh foods, and then Ayurvedic foods, then raw, then superfood and medicinal mushrooms, and now I have investigated high fat diets and reducing the carbohydrate load on my body, using really good fats and oils, at the same time doing high-intensity training and intermittent fasting and things are changing again.

It suits me to keep honing my relationship to what works, and as more and more research gets further inside nutrition I love it as it helps me drill down into what exactly might be going on. So Im trying to find the tests that will help me look at the ratio of fats, proteins and carbs particular to my ATP production. If you read my blog on www.thunderboltcoach.com you can keep up to date with what I find.

Summing this short chapter up I would say ... stay flexible, wise and adaptable.

Dogma has no place in diet.

THE PROBLEM IS YOUR MIND

"The problem is your mind." - **Dr Ye** *(my Chinese Doctor)*

At some point in your life, ill or not, you may have to consider whether your mind is your ally or your enemy.

It sounds like a ridiculous statement, but from my own experience and observing others, it is probably one of the truest things I have ever said.

If your mind is your foe, you are in trouble. It will destroy your life. It may destroy others lives also, but it will certainly destroy yours. You will never reach your potential, and you will never experience true health or happiness while your mind is untamed and unknown. Remember the saying, 'Heal Thyself and Know Thyself.' Knowing thyself means knowing the movement of your own mind, what kinds of things it says, what happens when it feels threatened, whether it really serves you, and bringing it into line.

Your mind and your emotions are working together. Everything is connected, so if your body is struck by illness, your emotions are also struck by illness, and your mind is also struck by illness. It is an imperative that we look into our own mind if illness strikes.

Consider this:

> *"Your mind is an instrument, a tool. It is there to be used for a specific task, and when the task is completed, you lay it down. As it is, I would say about 80 to 90 percent of most people's thinking is not only repetitive and useless, but because of its dysfunctional and often negative nature, much of it is also harmful. Observe your mind and you will find this to be true. It causes a serious leakage of vital energy,"*
> **- Elkhart Tolle.**

This 'vital energy' is what I call life force. Our life force is intrinsically connected to our mind, and of course our emotions.

What is Life Force?

When you hear that someone has a powerful or vibrant life force, what image do you conjure up in your mind? Probably you imagine someone full of life and vitality. They would be physically well and in their power. They would definitely be creative and they might exude success. That is life force.

Life force energy is the invisible energy that animates all living things. It is that which flows from the divine source into creation.

Life force is the natural flow of energy. It is what we are designed and intended to use as the energy for our lives. It is the intrinsic part of manifestation from spirit into matter, the bridge between the formless and form. In it's natural state it flows freely and gives life to that which it animates, and according to natural law, when life force begins to weaken and recede, so death arrives.

An abundance of flowing life force gives vibrant, creative life, and a weak, compromised life force brings sickness, decay and ultimately death. Disruption of life force is the energetic cause of dis-ease.

And here is the thing: life force is influenced by your thoughts and feelings. The quality of your thoughts leads to strength or weakness in your body. This is a truth easily overlooked in our search for healing. I cannot say this too many times.

Chronic illness, particularly, has its roots in the whole spectrum of life, from our lifestyle choices to our emotional wellbeing and the quality of our thoughts. This includes conscious and subconscious thinking. And anything to do with thinking means life force, because thinking influences life force.

You have the power to create health or create illness. You have the power to fully and consciously allow maximum life force to flow into and through your life, and your body. You also have the phenomenal power to block life force from flowing fully and freely into and through your life, and your body. One road may well take you to health, vitality and boundless energy. The other may take you to chronic illness, depression and an insufferable fatigue. That is the incredible power you have. You have a choice.

'The problem,' as my Chinese Doctor used to say to me, 'is your **mind**.'

What does this mean?

It means that thinking, particularly habitual thinking, has a direct influence over fundamental elements, organs and processes of your body, and that if there is a problem in the mind, no amount of good diet and healthy living will outweigh it. It is very powerful.

Research and latest science reveals that our genes are affected by our thoughts. But there is so much more. Our cells themselves are affected by our thoughts. Our immune system is affected by our thoughts, as is our digestive system. And now research suggests even our DNA itself changes shape depending on what we feel and think. The very building blocks of our body, our main protection system and the processes that keep things running smoothly are hardwired to our thoughts and feelings. Those thoughts and feelings are our life force.

On top of this, reports say the association between stress and dis-ease is as much as 85%. An estimated 121 million people world-wide currently suffer from depression. 50% of Americans say that they are increasingly stressed about their ability to provide for their family's basic needs.

Life force is obscured and blocked by anxiety and stress, and under the weight of work and family responsibilities, making money and buying into the modern life, anxiety and stress are very common. It is all about what you think about. Chronic thinking will inevitably lead to chronic dis-ease.

The problem is your mind.

So what can you do?

Positivity, love, gratitude, joy, creativity, laughter, enthusiasm and simply expecting the best possible outcome are some of the best medications you have at your disposal. But it is your responsibility to harness and mobilise your energy. It doesn't just happen by sitting back and doing nothing. This energy connects to your will. Your will and your life force are the same, and its possible for you to consciously feed them. There are two sides, but you can only feed one, either you feed negativity or your feed positivity. There is no fence to sit on.

Don't think yourself to an early grave.

My Chinese doctor found it incredible and insane that so many of his patients (all westerners), who develop symptoms, are so fear based that they jump to the most dreadful conclusions right from the start. He told me stories of patients who thought themselves to death through fear. If you read **Anita Moorjani's** book 'Dying to Be Me,' you will see that, from her profound experience, she discovered that her cancer had it's roots in fear, pure and simple. That's a heck of a thing to realise.

From my observations I would say that fear plays a part in every illness and dis-ease.

This is why it is so important for you, for me and for everyone, to do, say, think and feel things that feed life, love and joy. Making the choice to actively support life sends a message out to the universe that has repercussions the mind cannot understand, but can actively trust are for the good of one and all. Treat the world with suspicion and doubt and the world will reflect exactly that, you will live in a cold and hostile world. But show love, joy and enthusiasm for yourself and others and the world will mirror that, and you will live in a world that is much more favourable to healing. Try it for a while.

Suspicion, doubt, cynicism, and anger are all very acidic thoughts and emotions. They bring an acidity to the body. Love, joy, gratitude and compassion are very alkaline in their nature. They soften and heal. They bring this alkalinity to the acidic body and help heal it. Thoughts and emotions themselves are acidic or alkaline. They manifest in the body in this way, and thus are harmful or healing.

Create a momentum of enthusiasm in your life, whether you are well, sick or dying. So many of us live cautious, hesitant lives. We have been trained and conditioned to behave in certain ways, ways that mean we 'fit in' and 'don't rock the boat.' All this training is a double-edged sword. On one hand, it means we all live together in society. On the other hand, it kills our individuality, our inner authority and our wild untameable side. Imagine our old ancestors, the wild ones who hunted and gathered and survived outside by instinct and stealth, imagine them living in our modern houses and flats, and trying to work out how to fit in. Well, there is still a part of us that carries this wildness. It's connected to our life force. Sit on it too long and too hard and it will kill you.

Without any kind of outlet or expression, this wild side doesn't simply disappear. It lives inside us as a caged beast, depressed, lonely, unloved and neglected. It contributes greatly to the psychic cause of dis-ease.

So the first thing to do is say 'hi' to your wildness! You don't have to scream and run around naked (unless you want to)! I am talking about something more subtle and deep. This is a feeling, not something you need to do. It is a permission you give yourself, a decision and a commitment that you are not ruled by fear and you stand in your own authority. You consciously and persistently turn fear into excitement.

Positive life force is a big YES! It is the ignition of an inner fire. It is a statement of intent, and a statement of your intention to heal, even if that means just healing your fractured connection to yourself or God. Remember Einstein's words: "You cannot solve a problem using the same kind of thinking that created it."

My version reads:

You cannot heal disease with the same kind of thoughts that created it.

You need to choose to up-regulate the quality of your thoughts. I do not entertain self destructive thoughts for too long. I don't attach to them, I let them pass through. So when my mind starts complaining that, 'It's too hard, I'm too scared, why me?' etc (and I do still get these thoughts), I just bring awareness to them and allow them to drift across the sky like clouds, not hooking into them at all. And pretty soon they disappear over the horizon and are gone.

So raise the quality of thoughts. Opt to install a new thought program into your operating system. Upgrade to joy, gratitude, love, power, positivity and creativity. It is your life, it is your body, your thought and your choice. Own your thoughts, but don't let them own you.

Most people are running around with tape loops playing in their heads. The same thoughts go round and round, and most of these thoughts are inherited from other people, like mother and father and teachers. Claim your authority now, today.

Will it heal you?

It will help you in many direct and indirect ways. It will release energy, it will stimulate your immune system, relieve your adrenal glands and support your DNA. It will attract the positive attention of the universe and things may begin conspiring in your favour. Just do it without expectation, with no agenda other than to feel life pouring into your mind and body. It feels good. And if it feels good, it does good.

Life Force Meditation (10 - 15 minutes)

Spend some time sitting, or lying down, in a quiet comfortable space, alone, and supported by either calming music or the sound of nature. Begin by breathing softly and deeply, but neither pushing out or sucking breath in. Just relaxing every muscle, every digit, every limb, and relaxing attention and mind.

Drop everything to be in this moment.

Imagine your light astral body. Picture it in your mind. See it as a pulsating emanation of dazzling brilliant luminescent light, perfect in every way, radiating light and love in every direction. Be stunned at its beauty and divine perfection. In this astral body there is no sickness, no illness, no issues, no doubt, no toxicity, just the purest love you could ever imagine. The image is so powerful it makes you cry with joy, knowing this is the highest you, and that you are perfect.

Hold this image as long as you want and burn it deep into your heart. Never forget this moment.

Now, when you are ready, feel the sheer brilliant power and pure life force of this energy begin to stream down into your body as you lie or sit there. Feel it in your bones, your skin, your hands, feet, head, gut, everywhere. Feel it penetrate deeper and deeper into the cells of your body. Feel the pulsation of pure brilliance as it animates your being.

This is your essence, your life force. Allow it in, breathe it in with a big yes. Feel the light within this body.

It doesn't matter how broken, sick or damaged you are, allow this pure feeling of love to penetrate into the deepest parts of your body.

Tell your self you are perfect and brilliant as you are. Remind yourself you are love itself, you are pure consciousness spending some time in the dense realm of matter.

Remind yourself how positive, how powerful and how creative you are.

Remind yourself you are healed in this moment, and bring joy and love to this knowing.

Feel it as powerfully as you can with no self doubt or cynicism. Do the best you can, knowing you can return here any time you like.

When you feel satisfied you have done the best you can at this time, allow all thought to evaporate into the open sky of your consciousness and return to simply breathing gently in and out, and slowly bring yourself back to the present moment, and open your eyes.

Know that you can do this meditation any time you want. Do it every day for 21 days slowly, then return to it when you are called. But always remember that this is a truth and you can now picture and feel so easily the perfection that is you.

YOU GOTTA MOVE

I am a fan of exercise and do some sort every day unless I am too ill or having a day off to rest. But I wasn't always like this.

I stopped exercise when I was about fifteen, the same time my life imploded. There was absolutely no place for exercise in the life of a young traumatised hedonist. My body, in fact my health and well being, was on the lowest rung of my priority ladder. And it stayed that way until my mid thirties. As part of my attempt to 'get myself together' I started running. It took me at least a year to get anywhere near able to run properly. For the first few months I thought I would die each time I ran. I ran out of breath almost immediately, had absolutely no strength or endurance and was weak in all muscles. I got injured all the time, suffered from shin splints and pulled muscles, and most of all I felt defeated. But as you may know by now I am a persistent guy and I don't give up easily. I endured and slowly I improved in all areas. And I have said this before but I will say again, if I can do it anyone can!

Really, you don't know how far down I was.

For example, I used to share a flat with a tennis coach. He was super fit and agile. We lived on the second floor of a block, and one day we arrived home together. He bounded up the stairs two at a time as you might expect. I tried to do the same, ran out of steam after the first flight and crawled up the remaining stairs huffing and puffing. I had to lie down I was so out of breath. He was shocked! We were almost the same age, about thirty years old. And that was definitely a contributing factor to my chronic illness.

If you don't move it, at some point you gonna lose it.

Your body is a gift. It is the vehicle that carries consciousness while you are on the earthly plane. It demands your respect and care. That is your responsibility. Yet we have sacrificed this most basic of principles. Sometimes I see this as the age of sloth and lethargy, greed and narcissism.

A sedentary body, one that never moves or sits at the desk all day, particularly one that is ill or under par, needs to move if there is any hope of restoring system integrity. You will not do it without. We are designed to move around, to walk, trot, bend, stretch, breathe, jump, get tired, recover and do all this over and over again. That is what we did during our long evolution, before we all decided to sit down. We had no choice but to move, it was part of our survival and our nutrition. But sit down we did, and we never got up!

So we sit around all day, at desks, at friends, at the cinema, in front of the TV, at the restaurant. Our ratio of natural movement (as a society) dropped during the 20th Century, and our eating habits became increasingly more toxic. And the technological revolution has increased the burden, because now everyone who works in an office sits behind the screen all day.

So we invented exercise!

Looked at from a certain angle, exercise is a manufactured way of returning us to what we are designed to do naturally. Whenever I exercise I'm mimicking nature. How many overweight and out of shape wild animals do you see? None. The only animals you ever see overweight are the ones who come into contact with humans, like dogs, and the ones who are, sadly, caged and forced to live like prisoners.

Animals move around. They do not exercise.

Reassessing our understanding and re-framing it gives us some leverage when we meet our resistant body, emotions and mind. When many people think of 'exercise' they become reluctant and stubborn. How about just 'being natural?' What about the wild Indigenous Amazonian tribes? Do you imagine they exercise? What would they do, rebounding? Tree-swinging? Running! There is no need to exercise when the connection to nature is so strong.

But modern we are (although I do wonder sometimes), and so we replace the natural way with exercise. This separated movement from our natural way, we sat down, introduced processed food and thus created obesity, sloth, laziness, reluctance and ambivalence. It is a cultural phenomenon, and one that must be seen and overcome for wellness to thrive.

If people were lazy, slothful and reluctant during our ancient ancestor days, they would have died. They would have starved or frozen. Maybe they did anyway, but what I'm really saying is they didn't have any option. Animals in the wild, and indigenous tribes do not have an option, it's in their nature and in their survival instinct.

To survive (eat) you need to move (exercise). That connection has gone. Now the equation reads: To survive (eat) you need to get in your car and drive to the store (exercise).

Some of the problems

Desk sitting increases gut disorders, including bowel cancer, by a marked degree. IBS, IBD and all digestive issues can be impacted by sitting too long.

Desk sitting is also associated with a whole host of other chronic issues, from osteoporosis to diabetes, obesity, heart disease and early death. A lethargic and sedentary lifestyle contributes to chronic disease, of that there is no doubt. And of course chronic disease can happen even if you exercise but moving the body energy is one of life's core principles.

Look at children, they move all the time. They run, jump, bend and crawl. Sadly the technological age has even swallowed them, and many kids now spend their time in artificial light on play station and computer. Young people are weaker boned, more prone to illness, more depressed, more chronically sick and more medicated than at any time in history.

> *As I write I have just seen a post on Natural News Health site reporting that three quarters of 17 - 24 year olds in the US are not eligible to join the military because they don't possess the fitness or cannot meet basic requirements. It's frightening.*

So, no matter what state of health you are in, unless you are flat out bed-ridden, *you gotta move!*

Really, you can do whatever inspires you or excites you but move. 30 minutes a day, every day, move your bits.

Rebound, walk, run, skip, hop, do yoga or tai chi, dance, swim or cycle. It doesn't matter what you do, it just matters that you do.

Your lymphatic system cannot move toxins from your body unless you help it. Your blood has a pump, the heart, but your lymph system, and there is more lymph fluid than blood, has no pump. It relies on movement to keep it moving. It is a sticky, mucosal fluid prone to stagnation. And it is the lymph system that is partly responsible for moving and expelling toxins and waste from the cells. That's a pretty serious job that it gets very little help with, unless you move your body. And the movement it loves best is an up and down movement. Hence rebounding arrived.

I hope you know what a rebounder is. It's a mini trampoline. You can use it indoors or outside. A lot of research has been done on the benefits of rebounding when NASA looked at it as a possible solution for astronauts who lose up to 15% of their bone and muscle mass after only 14 days in zero gravity. The results were conclusive. Rebounding exercises the entire body without excess pressure on the feet and legs. There is less exertion on the heart, and you get more benefit with less oxygen. They also found that the acceleration and deceleration of rebounding provides benefits on the cellular level not available with other exercise.

The benefits are:

- It boosts lymphatic drainage and immune system function.
- It helps with digestion and elimination.
- It strengthens the skeletal system and increases bone mass.
- It helps oxygen circulate.
- It helps build a strong core.
- It increases oxygen to the brain.
- It improves muscle to fat ratio.
- It is good for balance and stability.
- *It's easy, you can do it when it's raining, and its fun!*

You can start with 5 minutes a day, just standing on it and getting used to the motion, and simply build up from there. You will not regret this. And once you are hooked you will love your rebounder. The only other point I would say is, don't buy the cheapest. Pay a little extra and get a good quality one with great bounce. It will serve you well.

Of course there are many other sorts of exercise that will work. If you cannot rebound, then walk for 30 minutes each day. And walking means walking at pace, not strolling. Put some effort into it, do some hills and feel it in your body. Breathe in the air deep into your lungs (providing you are not in a town centre)! And feel the light on your skin. Being outside and walking or running not only exercises the body, it also gets vital Vitamin D onto the skin. Research into Vitamin D is finding that low levels are seriously linked to all sorts of chronic diseases, including cancer. And covering oneself with unnatural suntan oil makes this worse. I have found that eating a high raw diet with fresh vegetables, lots of green leaves and coconut oil, protects the skin against most sun.

For myself, I like running. I used to run long distances, but have changed now to enjoy High Intensity Interval Training (HIIT). Burst training, as it is known, is fast and powerful, trains the body to burn fat, increases human growth hormone and is a quick and efficient way to upscale health.

But if you like cycling, rowing, swimming, gymnastics or dancing, these are excellent ways to shift energy and move the body.

Movement is the nature of life. When it is absent, energy becomes sedentary. Sedentary is not stillness. Sedentary is when something that should be moving is not. Look at the river. It is supposed to flow. When it flows it keeps clean and, providing it is not polluted upstream, it maintains it's fresh aliveness, is oxygenated and has life force. But if that same river is prevented from flowing it stagnates, and then something very different happens. It stops being oxygenated, life begins to disappear and things die in it and around it. It has no life force and we are repelled by it. We know something is wrong with it, it smells of decay and death.

I'm afraid this is not so dissimilar to us. Our energy is the same. It has to move through us. Exercise moves this energy. If the energy does not move through us, we have the same tendency as the river. Stagnation happens and entropy begins. Temporary entropy is ok, but chronic entropy is fatal.

If you have voices in your head that say you cannot do any exercise, I refer you to the previous chapter 'The Problem is Your Mind,' and if you are experiencing lots of stuck energy in your body I refer you to the chapter on healing your emotions. Get the energy moving. Activate your power, mental, emotional and physical power.

Note: I want to add a personal note here. I simply cannot convey to you how good it feels to be relatively fit, as I am these days. When I look back at how I was when I was in my twenties and thirties I shudder. I had so little energy in my body and in my emotions. I lived on borrowed energy, borrowed from stimulants and stress. It was never going to sustain. It can't sustain beyond a certain age, and then we really notice it. Now I have endless energy, I get no dips or spikes and feel very even. It has helped my sleeping habits and calmed by mind and emotions. It is a very grounding and stabilising force in my life, it gets me out into the world and into nature. Feeling fit is such a bonus in life.

And everyone can do something. Whatever it is, do it.

LIVING A NOBLE LIFE

"No matter how careful you are in choosing your food, know that you will obtain only mediocre results if you omit the most important thing - that is, making goodness the foundation of your life. If you do not respect each living being, if your thoughts are not pure and elevated, if a high ideal does not guide you while excluding all negative thoughts and feelings, you will introduce poisons into your body."

"To avoid that, send grateful thoughts, when you eat, to all of the beings, to the plants, to the elements, to the forces that take part in maintaining your existence. The awareness of the grandeur of life, and the sentiment of gratitude that you will feel filling up your heart with a vivifying warmth, will contribute to the development of everything great and noble that you receive," - **Beinsa Douna** *(1864-1944) Bulgarian Essene Master and musician.*

Beinsa Douna, otherwise known as Peter Deunov, has been the source of inspiration to Wayne Dyer, the famous motivational speaker/author, for many years. Wayne has, in the last few years, been on a very deep journey when he developed leukaemia. It's fascinating to hear him talk about illness from such a positive spiritual perspective. He offers an unshakeable belief that we affect the physical world with our thoughts and energy. He also takes action to support health in his body. But he does not indulge in any negativity at all! It is quite amazing to hear someone just so positive talking about very tough experiences. And I would say to you, if you are healing, get inspired all the time. Find books, audio recordings, use the internet, and friends who pull you up to a higher level of inspiration. It really works. It ignites your inner flame of right desire. Other people give you confidence and reassurance that you are not alone. Other people's stories are heroic. Everyone climbs the mountain at some point in their lives. Some come down and tell the story of how they did it. It doesn't mean you don't have to do it, and it doesn't mean you have to copy them, it just means it is possible, and that is enough to keep you going when it gets tough.

In order to steer our personal and collective ships through and beyond the turbulent waters of the current toxic chaos and dis-ease, we have to raise our own vibration and lift ourselves up to a new level of being. There is no other way. This is the essence of living a noble life.

A noble person cares deeply about all aspects of their own life and the lives of others and the planet. They care about the environment and the creatures who also walk this earth. They cause as little harm as possible, and do as much good as they can. Their word, thought and are congruent with the highest moral and ethical values, and they are deeply spiritual and humble beings, whose every moment is infused with love. This is about lifting one's personal integrity to a new high and living from that place. It lies within all of us to do this, yet we have traded in a life of depth and wisdom for one of acquisition and superficiality.

The Global Imperative

We are faced with Great Change. Everyone can feel it, consciously or unconsciously. Our times are intense, dramatic and changeable. Since the turn of the century we have witnessed the escalation of war, greed, terrorism, spying, Big Pharma and Food Inc. The weather is insane, countries and economies are going bankrupt, politicians seem scurrilous and driven by hidden motives, and hundred of millions of people are chronically sick simply because of the food they eat. The sea, the sky and the earth are dying, and the barbarity that humanity now inflicts on animals for the sake of its food is unimaginable. This is the face of collapse. Or maybe it is the face of *transformation!*

We simply cannot go on doing what we are doing, hoping that things are going to be all right. We cannot stick our heads in the sand any longer. But this is the thing:

> *The world will only be lifted to a higher plane of consciousness when each of us lifts ourselves to a higher plane of consciousness.*

It cannot be any other way. And, as the Masters, Saints and Prophets have said since time immemorial, the way is **love**.

The wave of divine fire is coming, we already feel it. It is beginning to burn each of us, in our lives, our dreams, our emotions and in our relationships. The fire will become more intense. It is a cosmic cleansing of all that is toxic, in us, in our society, on our planet and in our universe. If we are prepared for this fire and we accept it and allow it to purge and transform us, all will be well. If we resist and stay on the level of fear, we may be doomed to live in a state of perpetual fear for the rest of our lives. Choosing love and harmony now is the only answer, and living that as a reality day to day.

That means living by these 6 principles:

- Nourishing the body with simplicity and natural foods.
- Doing no harm.
- Taming greed and addiction.
- Living a heart based life with gratitude and love.
- Developing spiritual wisdom and peacefulness.
- Living a life of service.

As Peter Deunov says, *"A new culture will see the light of day, it will rest on three principal foundations: the elevation of woman, the elevation of the meek and humble, and the protection of the rights of man."*

There is going to be a new way, a new civilisation, that grows out of the remains of this one. Our current way has grown old and corrupt, it is morally bankrupt, and needs to be terminated. Nature itself is terminating it. And although it seems like the worst thing that could happen, as I have been pointing out during the whole book, things that appear to be 'bad' at first, tend to be the things that bring the greatest gifts.

But it means surfing the waves and opening to the principles now, today, in this moment, and tomorrow. Don't wait! It will be too late tomorrow.

This is the time to expand your mind and open your heart. It is the time to think more deeply and consider the real nature of your life and your purpose. It is the time to remove all that is unloving and gross. We are all poisoned in our bodies, hearts and minds, and only great purification of this poison will allow us through the gates of the next wave of humanity.

In the same way we can choose to see the events in our individual lives, the ones that arrive uninvited and take us by surprise, as burdens or blessings, we can choose to see the events unfolding in the world. We are scared of instability, so we would rather stick with a world that is driven by greed, inhumanity and rape of the earth, than gamble on massive change. But gamble we must, even if it hurts.

It is time to step out of the comfort zone and live our truth proudly and humbly.

Change of the entire hologram

There is not one area of the Universe that is not being changed and upgraded. And this is where you have an impact and a choice. You can stay as you are, or you can align yourself with cosmic forces and upgrade your cellular intelligence. Your cells are designed to absorb cosmic intelligence. They are antennae that are tuned in to the universe. But our toxic load clogs up the receptors on the cells and prevents them receiving this information. This information is vital to our freedom on earth and spiritual connection to the bigger galactic picture. Without this connection we are as prisoners, shut off from our true source of nourishment. Your cellular intelligence relates with the invisible world 'out there.' And thus the detoxifying and nourishing of your cells reconnects them to the cosmic source. Not only does it create physical health and well being, remove dis-ease and its symptoms, but it rewires you into the universe and divine intelligence. This is one of the most powerful ways you can upgrade your entire life and prepare for massive global change.

The Challenge

When the world around you is full of hate, greed, fear and corruption, **can you stand in the vibration of love**?

When your health is undermined and demands you take greater and greater responsibility, **can you stand in the vibration of love**?

When your house is washed away and your possessions lost, **can you stand in the vibration of love**?

If your body is taken from you by another's hand or dis-ease, **can you stay in the vibration of love?**

Can you say, like the great teacher and sage Krishnamurti said when asked what made him different from everyone else, '**I don't mind what happens.**'

That is the ultimate aim of my life, to reach profound peace, love and compassion for all living beings, and I hope it may become your aim also.

NEGATIVITY

A few words about dealing effectively with the influence of negativity is necessary.

Before I start let me make it crystal clear I do not, and have never, allowed other people's negativity to stop me doing anything. If I have been influenced by anything negative, it has been my own mind. That is slightly different. But this is about what we choose to surround ourselves with and the impact it has, and our personal responsibility therein.

We are porous beings and easily influenced by others. If we have any doubts within us about ourselves they are easily exploited, consciously or unconsciously, by others.

Many people have our best intentions at heart. That is at least what they say. And people are 'pack-like,' they tend to stick together and believe the same thing as each other. Not necessarily because they absolutely know it to be the truth, but because it is something they have been told is the truth and they have believed it.

And they will defend it until their dying breath.

...se people will include your family and your ...iends, professionals and people you innocently meet as you go through life.

I have encountered all this and I find it easy to shrug off their concerns and advise. I am extremely cautious, even allergic to, unsolicited advise. I gave up caring what people think or say long ago.

But you may still have an ear open to them. And their advise may steer you in one direction or another.

When you are ill you are vulnerable. Everything changes when you are ill and part of you becomes very open. This part needs protecting. There is no need to close it down. Just protect it.

Be very aware of what is happening around others. If you are ill you must be extra aware because you are in a highly vulnerable and easily influenced place. And the people around you will be scared, the closer they are to you the more scared they will be. They will be scared for you AND scared for themselves.

If you start talking about healing, alternative medicine, emotions, the mind and spiritual aspects of the whole journey, some of those people will freak out and think you have gone mad.

There have been lots of reported cases recently of women who have pulled their children out of hospital care and run off with them to seek radical and unorthodox 'natural' treatments. On the whole these women have been lambasted by the press and the conventional medicine institutions. When any of us steps out of the box we cause a stir. When we (or our loved ones) are sick, this stir can be profound and passionate.

When I signed myself out of the care of the hospital and walked bravely out of the building, the consultant looked at me as though I was insane and neglectful. He had all the authority, the knowledge and the arrogance of a man who was totally and absolutely sure he was right and everyone else was wrong. As it has turned out he was wrong. But according to convention and the rules of the game I should have listened to him and been completely guided by him. If I had been surrounded by the pressure of a family, and less of a rebel than I am I could quite easily have surrendered by authority, and I would not be here today writing this.

So be aware. Be very aware. Stand in your authority. Get an advocate who agrees with you. Seek independent counsel. Get many opinions. If you don't agree with your doctor's diagnosis, find another doctor who can give a second opinion. Your life may depend on it. Find sympathetic others. Join social media groups who believe what you do. Find allies, they are out there somewhere.

Surround Yourself with Positive People

Particularly if you are ill, but generally in life anyway, lose people who are constantly negative. The chances are you cannot save them, change them or fight them. Negativity is powerful. The energy it has seeks to draw everything else towards it and negate it.

...y surround yourself with people who support you or pull you up to a better place.

Negativity is like a black hole. It spins and spins and draws things towards it. It feeds on everything it devours. Think abut Eckhart Tolle's description of the pain body and how it has to feed on others, well it's the same thing. The black hole of negativity draws everything into it.

When you are going on the healing journey you simply do not need this. Of course you need to develop critical thinking. Clarity of mind and logical thinking are essential components of being well. But so is being positive, trusting your instincts, taking alternative natural measures, and demanding support.

Lift yourself up, and you will lift others. Drag yourself down, and you will try and drag others down.

Get Real, Not Happy

I am reminded of this because of Gabor Maté who has talked about falsely happy people who are confused as to why they get cancer. Many people say, 'I am always happy and have no idea why I got sick?' and he said, 'It's because your happiness is not real, it is a mask you wear. You have to let the dark in and deal with it, and everyone has darkness, it is part of being human.'

I would add, it is about being real not being happy. Being real opens us to allow everything. Allowing everything in means we have to deal with the negativity that lives inside us, and we have to take responsibility for our pain, for the hurt we have caused others, for our fear and for all the times we have turned away from love. There is hurt inside us. Until we are fully awakened there is always some hurt, some pulling away from life. I have met some incredibly happy people and most of them are extremely sad and depressed. They just wear a big fat mask to fool others and themselves.

ARISE WOUNDED HEALER!

In the Greek Myths, Chiron was a wise Centaur (half man, half horse, physician and healer). One night he was accidentally wounded by a poisoned arrow from Hercules' bow. Because he was immortal, Chiron was destined to live forever with a wound that would not heal, cursing him to eternal torment.

In his quest for a cure, he learned the great art of healing others, which brought some measure of solace but never healed his wound.

It is December 27, 2014. We have been in California for 3 months.

It has been a full year of birthing this book. It started in Goa, India, and finished in California, USA. I only picked up the book again two weeks ago and decided to finish it. The last few months I actually decided it was not good enough and I was going to start again, again! The journey of writing has led me to many places deep within myself, and challenged me time and time again. There have been moments I have felt completely aligned to my writing and very much 'in the flow,' and then other days when I felt woefully inadequate and on the verge of giving up. My health experiences have followed suit, from feeling so vibrant and unstoppable, to feeling very ill as though I was going to die. I have had all my symptoms come and go, haunting me and triggering thoughts of 'Who am I to be writing a book about my health journey, I'm not even healed!' But after much persistence and refusal to give in, I have finally concluded, '*Who am I NOT to be writing a book*!'

I was waiting to be perfect, hoping that one magnificent day the trumpets would sound and I would be able to announce, 'I am healed, world, now I can take my place!' It has been an unconscious thought that has limited me, probably all my life. Until I have discovered it in the last few days. It manifests as unworthiness and the thought of not being ready or up to the task. In a word, its bullshit. Humanity is, and has always been, obsessed by the idea of perfection and imperfection. It runs like a river through the main religions and it lurks deep down in the unconscious of each of us. It's what the great fall of Man is all about. It's big, and its nasty. And unobserved it can rule our lives. I have been a slave to it for many years. It is called the seeking of perfection.

So I have finally arrived at a place of acceptance that the apparent imperfection of things *is the perfection*. It is the mind that tells us we are not perfect and whole as we are, and the mind, as we know, is a cunning and demanding fox. It demands attention and feeding, and 'trouble' is what it feeds on. It cannot devour the perfection of the silent, peaceful, open heart, for there would be nothing for the mind to do. It would cease to exist. So it has to create division and separation. As long as you and I are searching for answers, searching for perfection, the mind is happy. At some point in the journey you simply have to stop listening to the doubting voice and say, 'I am perfect and I am here.'

Everyone carries a wound. Waiting to heal these wounds before you share your self with the world, as we have seen, is a futile task. You may never be ready. You already are ready. And the wound itself is your gift. It is your teacher and your doorway to depth, wisdom self knowledge and self love. He who knows and accepts himself teaches others to do the same.

Chiron teaches us that we are all healers when we embrace our wounds as gifts and share ourselves with humanity. The gift of individuality is that everyone is special and each carries a unique blessing to share with others. Find it and share it and you will experience joy. Hide it or deny it and it will only hurt you.

Trees in the Forest

You can walk the world with your wounds, and of course seek healing, but never let these wounds create limitation and self doubt. You are perfect, wounds and all!

Recognizing that our life's experiences create our uniqueness and individuality gives us the freedom to be creative. They make us, us. Like trees in the forest, we each grow with our twists and turns, our gnarly bits and grooves. But we are all growing in the same forest, and we are all reaching and growing towards the same light.

In fact, sharing of ourselves enables us to integrate our own wounds, it elevates them to a divine level. Our individual healing is intrinsically wrapped up with our service to others.

We cannot truly heal our wounds until we help others heal theirs.

Ram Dass tells us that his Guru, Neem Karoli Baba said, when he asked him how to be happy,

"Love everyone, serve everyone, remember God, and tell the truth."

We are not islands separated by vast stretches of loneliness. We are part of the interconnected whole, and our lives are intrinsically interwoven with each other.

We are in relationship, whether we know it or not, and that means we cannot truly heal our own wounds until we offer ourselves in service to each other. How to cultivate integration of your wounds and turn them into gifts? I would say that the most profound insights and depth I have gathered is when I have spent time alone in deep contemplation. I have done this at home, but also I have been out into nature and spent time alone. In my time, I have spent a night on the top of a mountain in Wales, UK. I took a sleeping bag to keep warm and ensure I didn't die, and let people know I was there, but otherwise I was alone. It was absolutely normal until the sun began to go down, and then it changed dramatically! Nature took over and I have never felt the absence of humanity as profoundly as that night. It was as though night time on a mountain was not the human world at all. I felt a complete stranger there, and it brought up fear and deep aloneness. I just sat all night listening to the voices and wind of the magical mountain speaking to me, I prayed and I contemplated my life. I was so pleased to see the dawn and my friends arriving to help me down! Another time, I spent the night in a cave alone in deep meditation. Solitude allows us to develop our inner being, and from our inner being our creative and healing impulse arises.

Seek solitude and know yourself. Share openly your joy and humanity with others and they will bless you for it.

How you share your gifts and what they are is something the mind cannot tell you. It has to come from your heart. The mind is a wonderful servant and will serve you well once you know where you are going, but it will lead you a merry dance telling you to do this, or that, or the other.

Knowing your mission in life comes from your higher self, from intuition, from your dreaming self, from a calling. That is the power of spending time alone, it encourages intuition and deep self knowing. You may get a flash of inspiration and that sets your body and soul on fire with a resounding yes! If it's quickly followed by a BUT then you may be on the right track. If your intuition seems way too big to reach, or makes you feel scared or small, you might be on the right track. Remember, you don't have to be perfect, you are perfect in your imperfection, and the world needs you so badly to be the best version of yourself.

The point is that you can share who you are not what you do. You can share your humanity, your experience, your truth, your brokenness, and your love. Most of all you can share your humanity. Sharing this is so much more powerful than what you do. Be intimate all the time. Engage others all the time. Be vibrantly alive all the time. Doing this is defenceless and open. It is so powerful.

I don't mean your story, the 'poor me,' the endless justification for your sorrows, I mean the deepest truth of your being, the truth below the story, the love, the redemption, the learning. We teach each other through sharing our deepest truth.

Everyone is a healer, everyone is in service to everyone else. We are all walking the same path, and as Ram Dass said, "*We are all walking each other home.*"

Accepting and loving yourself as you are right now heals the wound of seeking perfection and transforms you into your creative self, unfettered by doubt and anxiety, and free to help others in your unique way.

Arise wounded healer!

RADICAL WELL-BEING

The only genuine response to illness I have found is to radically meet it in the fire of transformation. By meeting it fully we allow ourselves the opportunity for it to burn up that which is no longer serving us and to change those things that no longer work.

There are always things to let go of and change. Habits, addictions, beliefs, grudges, stories, fears and negative programs.

Illness is the perfect invitation to stop and take stock of your life. There might be no other way that you would make the radical changes your higher self, or maybe your soul, wants for you. So listen hard to the messages, read the signs, learn the language of illness and begin to make changes. Open a deep and intimate dialogue with your body and ask it what it wants you to do. Don't just tell it all the time 'I want you to mend and get back on with the job of transporting me around.'

Ask and listen.

Wait, and sometime, at some point, your body, your intuition, will tell you. And be alert to how your body communicates with you, it can be subtle or profound, it can be in dreams or hunches. It could come from the outside via someone else. But it will be there and you must develop the awareness to listen.

We are receiving this feedback from the Universe all the time, but we are so preoccupied with ourselves we fail to notice, we fail to hear the whisper and we blunder on. We live in a vastly intelligent symbiotic universe that communicates with us. But we shut off our receptors and think we are alone.

We are not alone, we never were. We are one with the vastness of things. Developing the awareness and wisdom to be able to listen and effectively respond is part of our true heritage. We were designed for this. The denial of our natural abilities, and the suppression of the lines of communication contributes to our alienation AND our suffering. So when illness graces you, grab the opportunity and jump. It could be the invitation of a lifetime.

I know there is great suffering in illness, and it doesn't always go the way we want it to go. Many times it might mean the body dies, or we have to endure years of pain and hurt. This I obviously do not wish on anyone. But refusing to see anything good, any redeeming aspects of what has happened keeps us locked out of the possibility of transformation. Transformation does not mean we will survive. Ultimately I am talking about who you really are, maybe I am talking to your soul. When you have managed to heal your fear of whether you live or die, you can actually meet death consciously and peacefully.

Meeting death consciously is the purpose of life. And you cannot meet it consciously until you are liberated into love.

Illness comes as a reminder of your mortality. It is a powerful visceral reminder that you are going to die. And it is that which terrifies us. And it is this terror itself we are being invited to transcend. Transcending the fear of death allows unconditional love to flood our heart and mind. When unconditional love becomes our dominant state of being it no longer matters whether we live or die. Ironically the possibility of physical healing improves considerably because love is such a powerful healing force miracles can happen.

Unconditional Love

All the miracles you have heard of came because they were bathed in unconditional love.

> *A miracle is nothing more than the physical manifestation of unconditional love.*

All the stories of Jesus healing the suffering of others point to one thing: unconditional love. This love is the birthright of each of us. The task of our karma, our experiences, and yes our illness, is to return us to the place of our birth, the state of unconditional love. Sadly we believe that unconditional love is the province of saints, sages and seers and not us. This is a myth.

We are born to innocence. We are conditioned to fear.

We know this state in our very DNA. It is our soul, our absolutely pristine state. It cannot be erased it can only be forgotten. And it lies in the heart of hearts of each one of us. And that means it can be remembered. It can be remembered not as a thought or a theory, but it can become a lived experience. As a theory it has no power, but as a living experience, an embodiment, it has power beyond measure. It has the power to heal others, to transform situations, it has the power to bring light where there is darkness and bring balm where there is great suffering. This is the power to heal the world. If ever we were to completely forget this one truth as a species we would vanish quickly.

When I ventured deep inside myself like a deep sea diver exploring the ocean floor, when I went beyond everything and everyone and I found myself on the bottom, below fear and rage, below everything I could name, I found love to be there waiting for me. It was there all along, silently and patiently inviting me to come home. Unconditional love is always there. Human experience is there to show us where it is not, and invite us to welcome it back.

"The more you are motivated by love the more fearless and free your actions will be." - **Dalai Llama**

This is what I mean by **Radical Well-Being**. Turning around and meeting illness head on and face to face. Being prepared to face anything, even one's death, consciously choosing love over fear, changing that which needs to be changed, digging out and dropping addictions and false beliefs, these are truly radical activities. The blessings they bestow are enormous and life changing. You will become a warrior of the heart and you will impact all those who are quietly suffering in helplessness. You can truly help no one until you yourself are healed. As I said in 'Arise Wounded Healer!' that does not necessarily mean you have to be cured or super healthy. It simply means your heart and your mind must have been transformed and purged of fear.

When you have become love you are home, and it no longer matters about the state of the body. This is the lighthouse from which others navigate their path. They see you and are guided to the shore. This level of love is vast and indescribable. It is the love the mystics dream about, and the poets write about, and the sages teach of. It is home.

CONCLUSION

Thank you for reading my book. I have tried to convey some inspiration that might help you, or someone you know, to lift their heads up in the face of difficulty. I have tried to get at least some information across that suggests all the help we need is available, sometimes directly and sometimes arriving through mysterious channels.

I have tried to offer hope in sometimes seemingly hopeless situations.

I have tried to show, through my own journey, that it is not hopeless.

I have tried to say that we are not alone when we step out from the crowd and go our own way. Many others are doing the same thing. It is a movement of people who are seeking to take power back, power over their own health and wellbeing, and lives. We are in danger of being suffocated by the very governments we elect to protect us.

I have tried to point you in the direction that might help, and show some of the obstacles that you may have to deal with.

I have tried to show that, at a certain threshold, the journey may even become your life's defining story.

It could turn out to be the greatest blessing you have received in life.

I have tried to show that we might be treating this whole illness thing in the wrong way by constantly waging war on it and denying it, suppressing symptoms and hating its presence.

I have tried to show that a fundamental shift of awareness could be the best thing we ever did for ourselves.

I have tried to inspire you about the power of detoxification, through Panchakarma or fasting.

I have tried to point you to becoming flexible and mature in your attitude to food, using raw food, healthy fats, and deeply listening to your body needs.

I have tried to say that if you are carrying sub conscious thoughts or toxic emotions, they will always get in the way of true healing and holistic health. They must be dealt with.

I have tried to say that love is the only true answer to every question, and fear is the opposite of love. Fear must be dealt with and removed from the organic system. If it runs rampant it will destroy.

And now, dear reader, it is down to you to do what you must do.

If ever you should need support my coaching facility may be for you. Look me up and bookmark my site. I would be honoured to work with you.

www.thunderboltcoach.com

PART THREE
USEFUL RESOURCES

USEFUL RESOURCES

21 things you can do right now to create better health!

These tips are brought to you by personal experience. I have used them all and tried them all. This is by no means the full list, but I guarantee that if you apply these guidelines within a month you will begin to notice the difference.

Bear in mind you may experience some detox reaction, particularly if you are eating a toxic diet (meat, dairy rich, chocolate rich, alcohol etc), but if you persist you WILL experience improved health.

And bear in mind also that if you experience any side effects or feel in any way ill please go to your Doctor and get a health check, if you think it will do any good.

1. **Scrape your tongue.** Buy a tongue scraper and every morning when you get up scrape the tongue and remove the excess mucus that has built up overnight. Scrape from the back of the tongue to the front,

removing all residue as you do it. Do this before you brush your teeth.

2. **Warm water in the morning.** Drink 2-3 glasses of warm spring water with squeezed fresh lemon every morning after brushing your teeth. This helps dilute the toxins, flush them out and settle the stomach.

3. **Take Wheatgrass every day.** Wheatgrass cleanses the blood, reduces blood pressure, increases red blood cell count, boosts metabolism, detoxifies the liver and removes heavy metals and other pollutants from the body. It is full of enzymes and very alkalising. It also heals the colon wall and can be used directly on the skin to heal cuts and burns. In addition, it rejuvenates cells, slows down the ageing process and makes you feel alive! If it is fresh, take a shot a day. If it is dried powder, one or two heaped teaspoons a day, you can mix in a glass of water or apple juice, or add to smoothies and salad dressings.

4. **Chlorella.** Chlorella is a micro-algae with the highest concentration of chlorophyll of all foods. It is the number one medicinal food for cleansing the blood and eliminating toxins, not only being able to remove accumulated digestive pollutants but also alcohol, pesticides, heavy metals and radiation. It cleanses the liver, the bowels and the tissues of the body. On top of this, Chlorella also greatly supports the immune system, destroys bacteria and viruses, and contains a mysterious but scientifically identified substance

called Chlorella Growth Factor which dramatically heals tissue and fights free radical damage. Not to mention it's extremely high protein content, vitamins (including all the B's), minerals, amino acids and very high concentration of RNA for cell repair!

5. **Spirulina**. Spirulina is one of the many kinds of blue-green algae that grow naturally all around the world. It has the highest concentration of protein of any food, is rich in vitamins (especially Bs), minerals, essential fatty acids, antioxidants, enzymes, phytonutrients and nucleic acids (RNA and DNA). It is said that you could live on Spirulina alone and get all your protein and nutrient needs! Spirulina is a powerful blood builder, immune booster, protector from free radical damage to the cells and remover of heavy metals in the body.

6. **Exercise 30 minutes each day**. There is overwhelming scientific evidence that people who lead active lifestyles are less likely to suffer from illness and more likely to live longer. Exercise not only makes you physically fitter, it also improves your mental health and general sense of wellbeing.

7. **Drink Fresh Juices**. Drinking fresh juices made from fresh veg (green) and ripe fruits is very good for you. Start the day with a juice.

8. **Start eating green vegetables**. Green vegetables carry Sun energy. They are literally alive! The raw

revolution is discovering that these green leafy veg are just the most nutritious healing foods that exist. What green veg? Kale, spinach, chard, pak choy, broccoli, zucchini, and salad leaves.

9. **Go organic**. Whenever possible choose organic food. That way you avoid harmful pesticides. Put organic as a priority. You need to give your body as much help as possible to create amazing health, it doesn't just happen by accident. So put organic top of the list.

10. **Stop the snacks**. If you must eat snacks, make them healthy! Eat goji berries and bee pollen, or a piece of fruit. If you absolutely must snack then keep it healthy.

11. **Chew your food**. A pilot study at Indiana State University found that mindfulness, including specific instructions to slowly savour the flavour of food and be aware of how much food is enough, helped to reduce eating binges from an average of four binges per week to one and a half. Chewing food fully aids in the proper transport of nutrients in your body. The benefits of your body getting all the nutrients it needs are endless. Digestion is directly linked to the health of our cells, and all parts of the digestion process are crucial to being healthy.

12. **Get some sunlight**. Sunlight on skin and eyes is going to help your health enormously. If you don't get enough Sun begin Vitamin D supplementation.

13. **Eat at regular times**. You don't have to be rigid about it, but while you are getting your health back in alignment it is a really good idea for the body to know when it is going to eat. When you are super healthy then you can eat when you want, but you won't want to. Until then become a regular eater. And don't eat your last meal too late. Go to bed empty. Leave 2 hours after your last meal before you go to bed. And the last meal of the day shouldn't be the biggest.

14. **Go to bed early**. In Ayurveda they say going to bed before 10pm is the best thing you can do, after that the pitta (fire energy) starts to rise, then second wind happens and you wake up. If you can get to bed early and sleep it's a good habit to get into.

15. **Get up early**. Rise early and meditate if possible. Get up with the sun, 5.30 - 6am. Do yoga, be quiet and reflective. It's a great start to the day and settles you into yourself before the business of the day begins.

16. **Drink less tea/coffee**. Caffeine drinks tax the kidneys. Habitual drinking of these drinks is not great. Make a conscious effort to cut down. See where it is not necessary but just habitual. Practice going without for a day and feel how it is in the body and mind. Do you find yourself craving the coffee? If so you have an addiction, and at some point you may need to deal with this. If you must drink coffee, find the best quality, freshest coffee you can, never have pasteurised milk or soya milk, and opt to use raw,

grass-fed butter and make bullet coffee. Look it up on the internet and try it out. It is incredible!

17. **Drink more water**. Are you drinking enough water? Fresh spring water? Statistics are showing that the majority of populations in the west have never been fully hydrated! The impact of not having enough water is big. Organ deficiency, weight conflict, toxic build up. Drink more water. Do not gulp water, sip it slowly throughout the day. This simple action will help with your overall hydration.

18. **Reduce alcohol**. Alcohol in absolute moderation would appear to be ok. Can you keep it in moderation? If you can, great. But let's address those of you that can't. In anything over the absolute minimum, it is very dangerous, destroys liver and creates havoc in your life. Cut it down or give it up. If you must then drink high quality wine. Most beer is laced with GMO wheat.

19. Remove **Wheat** and **Sugar**. To many health advisors these two products are simply the worst for your health. You only have to look at the research to see for yourself. Making an effort to reduce intake will pay you so many dividends you will never regret it. If you are one of the millions of people eating too much, then yes you will experience withdrawal symptoms if you give up. That is simply because they are addictive, and you may well be an addict. Wake

up and get conscious of the things you are addicted to, physically and emotionally, it could save your life.

20. **Cut out milk and dairy, unless it is raw.** Milk and dairy products are the worst mucus generators of all. They will seriously clog you up inside and are one of the chief culprits in the current illness epidemic. Loaded with antibiotics, herbicides, pesticides, and hormones. If you must have milk and dairy, ensure it is always unpasteurised and grass fed.

21. **Take care of your adrenals and kidneys.** The majority of people in modern society are suffering from some kind of adrenal exhaustion. If the adrenals are not working well, the kidneys are not working well, and you are in a state of exhaustion. And so you reach for things to give you energy. These stimulants give a short term boost but a long term crash. You will pay the price in the long term with chronic exhaustion and organ depletion. Nourish and support these two organs through nutrition and relaxation, through high quality water, and through regular deep and restful sleep.

22. **RELAX!**

Book list:

- Andreas Moritz, *Liver and Gallbladder Cleanse*
- Norman Walker, *Colon Health*
- Markus Rothkranz, *Health 101*
- Donna Gates, *Body Ecology Diet*
- Bruce Lipton, *Biology of Belief*
- Charlotte Gerson, *The Gerson Therapy*
- Barbara Wren, *Cellular Awakening*
- J. Wilson, *Adrenal Fatigue*
- David Hawkins, *Healing and Recovery*
- Robert Morse, *Detox Miracle Sourcebook*
- Dr V. Lad, *Ayurveda, the Science of Self-Healing*
- Robert Young, *PH Miracle*
- Gabriel Cousens, *Conscious Eating*
- Stephen Harrod Buhner, *The Transformational Power of Fasting: The Way to Spiritual, Physical, and Emotional Rejuvenation*
- Dr. Jeffrey S. Bland, *The Disease Delusion*
- Amoda Maa, *Radical Awakening: discovering the radiance of being in the midst of everyday life*
- Terry Wahls, *The Wahls Protocol*
- Kelly A. Turner, *Radical Remission*
- *Gospel of Peace of Jesus Christ*

- Nina Planck, *Real Food*
- Dave Asprey, *Bullet Proof Diet*
- Michael Pollan, *The Omnivores Dilemma*

Films:

- *Unacceptable Levels*
- *Fat, Sick and Nearly Dead*
- *Food Matters*
- *Food.Inc*
- *Simply Raw: Reversing Diabetes in 30 days*
- *Burzynski: The Movie part 1 and 2*
- *The Gerson Miracle*
- *The Beautiful Truth*
- *Super Size Me*
- *Hungry for Change*
- *Crazy Sexy Cancer*
- *The Future of Food*
- *A Delicate Balance*
- *Forks over Knives*
- *Fast Food Nation*
- *Earthlings*
- *SuperJuice Me*

For Inflammatory Bowel Disease and Gut Health:

- https://www.myosiaffiliate.com/ltygshoppe/redir.php?oid=1023_11
- https://im177.isrefer.com/go/healthygutorder/kaviji/
- http://www.drdavidwilliams.com/ulcerative-colitis-natural-treatments/
- https://www.youtube.com/user/DiverseHealthService/videos
- https://www.youtube.com/user/robertmorsend
- http://bodyecology.com
- http://paleoleap.com/eat-this-bone-broth/

If you enjoyed this book please join me
and like my Facebook Page at:
https://www.facebook.com/PowerofIllness

And check out the new website at:
http://thepowerofillness.com

Printed in Great Britain
by Amazon.co.uk, Ltd.,
Marston Gate.